"If you love language this is the book for you. Paola Golinelli is a beautiful writer, creating understanding through writing that is more like an impressionistic painting than a scientific tract, but with the insights and psychoanalytic heft that will satisfy anyone looking for greater understanding of our complex, always expanding profession. Her voice is lyrical and gentle, inviting the reader to join her rather than argue one into submission."

Fred Busch, Ph.D.*, author of* Creating a Psychoanalytic Mind *(Routledge)*

"With this remarkable collection of essays Paola Golinelli has given us an invaluable gift. With insight, sensitivity and extensive knowledge of her subject matter, she has effectively employed an analytic lens to illuminate the artistic experience in its many forms and dimensions. The heart of Golinelli's book is her analytic discussion of a number of memorable films, a discussion that both enhances our understanding and deepens our appreciation of these woks of cinematic art. The same can be said of her essay on writing and of her original observations on the experience of viewing a great painting. This is a book to read, reread, and to treasure."

Ted Jacobs*, Training and Supervising Analyst of the ApsaA*

"This book written by Paola Golinelli is the brilliant work of an analyst who brings psychoanalytic exploration in the vast field of culture. It is a sensitive study of human emotions when confronted with a work of art, painting, statue, or cinematographic image. *Psychoanalytic Reflections on Writing, Cinema, and the Arts* deals with the human experience of integrating the object, while incorporating in this experience the object's absence. With sensibility and insight Golinelli describes situations in which encounter with the beauty of an object and loss of the object alternate and co-exist in subjective experience. The author uses psychoanalytic tools to interpret the internal as well as the external world. It is applied psychoanalysis at its best."

Ilany Kogan*, Training and Supervising Analyst, Israel Psychoanalytic Society*

Psychoanalytic Reflections on Writing, Cinema, and the Arts

"Why are we so fascinated by beauty?" is a question many of us have asked ourselves, as have many who came before us. This book investigates the moment of ecstatic solitude in which everyone can experience emotions through films, works of art or natural phenomenon, when, even if for a "magic" instant, we feel "alive" and masters of our own Self.

Expanding from the author's personal experience, this book is a series of applied psychoanalytic essays on film, literature, and aesthetic pleasure. It explores the complexity of loss and mourning, destructivity, perversion, and revenge, as well as an exploration of what can facilitate transformation and how to lead a blocked healing process back to motion.

This fascinating and insightful book will be of interest to psychoanalysts, psychologists, teachers and students, and all those with an interest in psychoanalysis and the arts.

Paola Golinelli is a Training and Supervising Analyst of the SPI (Italian Psychoanalytic Society) and works in private practice in Bologna. She is a member of the IPA in Culture Committee.

PSYCHOANALYTIC IDEAS AND APPLICATIONS SERIES

Recent titles in the Series include

Transformational Processes in Clinical Psychoanalysis: Dreaming, Emotions and the Present Moment
Lawrence J. Brown

The Psychoanalyst and the Child: From the Consultation to Psychoanalytic Treatment
Michel Ody

Psychoanalytic Studies on Dysphoria: The False Accord in the Divine Symphony
Marion M. Oliner

Contemporary Perspectives on the Freudian Death Drive: In Theory, Clinical Practice and Culture
Edited by Victor Blüml, Liana Giorgi and Daru Huppert

Permanent Disquiet: Psychoanalysis and the Transitional Subject
Michel de M'Uzan

Psychoanalytic Work with Families and Couples: Clinical Perspectives on Suffering
Susana Kuras Mauer, Sara Moscona, and Silvia Resnizky

Narcissistic Fantasies in Film and Fiction: Masters of the Universe
Ilany Kogan

Psychoanalytic Reflections on Writing, Cinema and the Arts: Facing Beauty and Loss
Paola Golinelli

Psychoanalytic Reflections on Writing, Cinema, and the Arts

Facing Beauty and Loss

Paola Golinelli

Routledge
Taylor & Francis Group
LONDON AND NEW YORK

First published 2021
by Routledge
2 Park Square, Milton Park, Abingdon, Oxon OX14 4RN

and by Routledge
52 Vanderbilt Avenue, New York, NY 10017

Routledge is an imprint of the Taylor & Francis Group, an informa business

British Library Cataloguing in Publication Data
A catalogue record for this book is available from the British Library

Library of Congress Cataloging-in-Publication Data
A catalog record has been requested for this book

ISBN: 978-0-367-48251-0 (hbk)
ISBN: 978-0-367-48250-3 (pbk)
ISBN: 978-1-003-03885-6 (ebk)

Typeset in Times New Roman
by Taylor & Francis Books

To Davide

Contents

Series Editor's Foreword

***Psychoanalytic Reflections on Writing, Cinema, and the Arts: Facing Beauty and Loss*, by Paola Golinelli**

The Publications Committee of the International Psychoanalytic Association continues, with the present volume, the series "Psychoanalytic Ideas and Applications."

The aim of this series is to focus on the scientific production of significant authors whose works are outstanding contributions to the development of the psychoanalytic field and to set out relevant ideas and themes, generated during the history of psychoanalysis, that deserve to be known and discussed by present day psychoanalysts.

The relationship between psychoanalytic ideas and their applications needs to be put forward from the perspective of theory, clinical practice and research, in order to maintain their validity for contemporary psychoanalysis.

The Publication's Committee's objective is to share these ideas with the psychoanalytic community and with professionals in other related disciplines, so as to expand their knowledge and generate a productive interchange between the text and the reader. The IPA Publications Committee is pleased to publish *Psychoanalytic Reflections on Writing, Cinema, and the Arts: Facing Beauty and Loss* by Paola Golinelli.

In this book, Dr Golinelli has creatively gathered together a collection of essays on beauty and loss, revisited in a series of applied psychoanalysis on film, literature and the arts. Dr Golinelli's interest in exploring the links between beauty and loss begins with an exploration of the links of early interactions between the infant and the mother. The author focuses on the infant's experience of ecstatic beauty in the encounters with the mother ("terrible unexpected beauty"), which are accompanied by the loss of this joyful experience due to the other side of maternal love: her absence.

The author develops the idea that the experience of beauty provides a privileged access to understanding the meaning and value of life, it offers an escape from a lack of sense implicit in the experience of loss. Elaborating on this basic idea, the author explores the moment of blissful experience through films and works of art. An added contribution of this book is the author's ability to weave together the psychic processes involved in analytic work and in writing. It is worthwhile noting that Dr Golinelli's beautiful writing elicits the very positive and aesthetic experience that is the focus of her book.

There is little doubt that this book provides important insights into the understanding of the links between loss and beauty as well as the importance of art, literature and films in providing meaningful emotional experiences. One should be thankful to Dr Golinelli for her insightful and creative contribution. I am confident that this volume will be useful and of much interest not only to the psychoanalytic reader worldwide, but to anyone interested in psychoanalysis, cinema and the art.

Gabriela Legorreta
Series Editor
Chair, IPA Publications Committee

Preface

A dedication

It was my father who gave me the gift of being enchanted by art. He was the first to take me to the cinema, opening the door to the discovery of one of the little, great joys of life. Then, that gift was reinforced by the passion of my teachers who equipped me with tools for historical and critical understanding.

It was only many years later, when I encountered psychoanalysis, that I became aware of the meaning I had found in the novels I had "devoured" during my adolescence, in the paintings whose colours had enthralled me and which I loved intensely without realizing their emotional weight, and in the films whose every scene was engraved in my memory and which I could watch over and over ad infinitum so that I could experience those emotions again. All this was without understanding that all those metaphors, all that visual and verbal heritage was waiting to find meaning.

It was only when I encountered psychoanalysis that I realized I was, step by step, uncovering the tools with which I would become more aware, and less fearful of my emotions, of my affections, and of remembering that they are human emotions and affections, even if not all humans are able to name them or to tolerate that awareness.

Thanks to the wise calm of my analyst, this encounter allowed me to assess the access routes to the unconscious which I – a Hitchcock film lover – had feared, like I might fear a monster with seven heads. It was something one shouldn't get too close to, on pain of terrible revelations and unsettling encounters.

Our love for things is born at home, in the family in the first years of life, and often has a significant oedipal component. This is certainly true for me, because my father loved cinema and he took me to it very early on; this was true also because, basically, he would not have otherwise been able to go himself. At that time in fact, having a babysitter was not common and, even if something of that kind did exist, my parents would certainly not have been able to afford it. So, if they had not taken me with them, they wouldn't have been able to go themselves. For my father, giving up films was simply impossible.

I have often wondered what his life would have been like without cinema. Certainly, it would have been sadder, flatter. In fact, my father was a dreamer, and cinema had furnished him from youth with a never-ending source of dreams. He was willing then to make economies on a modest apprentice's salary so that he could go to see the silent comedies of the day.

Perhaps cinema did not teach him much, as Tullio Kezich[1] says, even if I am not so sure of it, but it certainly did make him friendlier and more agreeable to the people around him. What is more, I am sure that it comforted him in the face of much fatigue, the suffering life imposed, and the anxieties he experienced with work. For this reason, he never did forgo it, except perhaps towards the end of his life. Certainly, when cinema held no more appeal for him it seemed to us to signal the unavoidable truth: that his time was near.

He loved all films, whatever their genre – drama, comedy, western, historical – but he had a special predilection for American films. His love for the musicals and comedies of Ginger Rogers and Fred Astaire was such that – as Kezich wrote somewhere (but I cannot remember where anymore) – he too, when their films ceased to arrive in Italy, knew that something serious was about to happen.

Not even the war stopped him from going to the pictures, however. He loved the *telefoni bianchi* and everything that fascist cinema produced in those years of autarchy and then of war. He had some favourites among both actors and films, whereas he was not so well-versed on the directors, and that was one of the ways he influenced me. I too, up to a certain age, knew the actors and the titles of the films, but I omitted directors. It was as if the fact that they did not appear in any scenes, and therefore did not give any visible contribution to the beauty and the spectacle, made them insignificant in our eyes.

The great silent films, Charlie Chaplin and the silent comedies, had enriched his childhood and adolescence with dreams. They had the power to unleash uncontrollable laughter even in his later years. So true was this that at one time he was forced to leave the theatre, because his laughing had turned into a sort of debilitating, convulsive coughing fit. His laugh was unmistakable among all the others, and it could fill the theatre with its sonorous ring and child-like levity. At the cinema the child in him came out, that child which had had to take on adult-like responsibilities far too soon. His need to laugh, to lighten up, just like a child who has been taken away from playtime too often, would take over and explode with a kind of gaiety which always characterized him. He was famous in our family for his likeability, his tendency to get distracted or to change his mood suddenly when simply reminded of a scene from a movie or an aria from a beloved opera. Opera was, in fact, his other greatest love.

One film in particular, perhaps, struck him with particular force: *La Nemica*[2] (1952) with Elisa Cegani. He would tell me about it with great feeling, as something which had left its mark on him. It was as if it had given him the cinema version of the same fraternal jealousy he felt for his older brother and for his sister – the beautiful Aunt Maria who, according to him, was their mother's favourite. He was very handsome himself, in some of the photos from his youth, in his Sunday best, brown suit with white stripes and his tan beret. That is what my mother must have thought, when she saw him walk by on Sunday afternoons on the way to go dancing in town. She started waiting to see him pass on weekdays too, on his bike, whistling; but people said he was the secret fellow of an older woman, single, maybe a widow, beautiful nonetheless and different from the others, and – above all – cashier at the cinema, where he had met and courted her. Or maybe she had courted him. Who knows?! Anyway, it had to do with cinema!

Notes

1 In his biography of Federico Fellini, the film critic, Kezich, writes, "Fellini's opera exercises one of the rights of the art, and that is not to teach anything, but to be able to make everything around us friendlier."
2 *La Nemica* (1952), directed by Giorgio Bianchi.

Acknowledgements

I am indebted to some very dear friends and colleagues for having got me to the end of this book. First among these is Warren Poland, for his ever-generous suggestions and for his patient support.

I thank Cordelia Schmidt Hellerau and Fred Busch, because the first idea for this book was born one evening while vacationing in Castellina in Chianti (Tuscany), during a dinner cheered by excellent food, good wine, and their precious company.

Of course, that evening Stefano Bolognini was present too – life companion and companion in psychoanalysis, to whom my special thanks are due for his affectionate patience and for our daily, rich exchange of ideas, impressions, and dreams.

A special thank-you goes to the translators Gina Atkinson, Aldo Grassi, Paola Merlin Baratter and Audrey Ellis Saracco for their careful and precious work.

In closing, I would like to thank the journals and publishers who granted permissions to reprint: *International Journal of Psychoanalysis, Psychoanalytic Quarterly, Rivista Italiana di Psicoanalisi*, the websites of the Italian Psychoanalytic Society (SPI) and the International Psychoanalytic Association (IPA), and Routledge.

Introduction

Why facing beauty and loss?

I consider beauty and loss to be closely linked themes in an analytic sense, starting with Freud's own writing in *On Transience* (1915). They are tightly tied in the same way in individual development, from the recognition of mother's face, her breast, and the smile in her eyes – the first elements of encountering the object. The ability to keep the mental image of that founding experience alive links to the possibility of calling it up in a hallucinatory way, to create it where needed (Winnicott, 1971), and thus affirm the supremacy of eros over thanatos. The subject's ability to symbolize, which at first bridges the gap between concrete and abstract and which allowed mental survival, comes back on stage at every new encounter and forces us to perform again the complex mental operation which re-constitutes or constitutes the object, integrating and incorporating in it the object's absence, and affirming the object and its negation all at once. Every time this occurs, we must again face the question of how much we can tolerate the unknowableness of the object, of its otherness. Thought is, in fact, an imperfect reproduction of the object, and so it is destined to frustrate, thanks to that irreducible difference between concrete presence and absence which will forever escape the subject's own control. The individual's various defence and survival strategies are based on that gap, as is the feasibility of carrying out analytic therapy.

My subtitle, "Facing Beauty and Loss" might seem cryptic and enigmatic. I believe, however, that it can give direction at that fork in the road between pathological outcomes and creative developments, where one can go toward a full-blown disease or toward a sublimated form, when put before the experience of encountering or facing the object, with its "terrible" and unexpected beauty. Beauty is the privileged access to understanding the meaning and the value of life, it leads to truth. This can save us from the lack of sense, and the absence of meaning – elements which connote loss and trauma.

Perhaps no one has defined what "beauty" is better than Keats (1817) in his famous lines:

When old age shall this generation waste,

Thou shalt remain, in the midst of other woe

Than ours, a friend to man, to whom thou say'st,

'Beauty is truth, truth beauty,' – that is all

Ye know on earth, and all ye need to know.

Being before a work of art, painting, statue, or cinematographic image can evoke many reactions. In that moment of ecstatic solitude, which rapidly dissolves but which probes in the deep and in the uncanny, the subject can experience very strong emotions: they can feel enchantment or refusal; they can feel lost or they can fall prey to Stendhal's syndrome (Magherini, 2007). They can, however, also feel they are in contact with a hidden or "forgotten" part of their Self, and leave this experience with a new acquisition. Ogden (1989) described this by talking about the autistic-contiguous position, that which together with schizo-paranoid and depressive ones alternate in more mature subjects and can, on the other hand, be unlikely or impossible to experience in states of disease. Meltzer (1988) talked about "the apprehension of beauty" in relation to the maternal image: the mother's face fascinates the infant and leaves the infant feeling ecstatic, but at the same time, it exposes the infant to the other side of maternal love – to her distancing herself, to her ambivalence.

When I started thinking about possible titles for this book, I had two in mind: "Facing Beauty and Loss" and "Between Beauty and Loss." Ultimately, I prefer the first one, because the second refers to the experiential feeling of being caught in a paradox: which path to follow, the one towards creativity or the one towards pain … And are they inevitably the same path? And where do they finally part ways? A preposition like "between" does not have the power to call up the emotional immediacy of the verb "to face", which was what I want to underline.

Films, literature, art – they can bring up in us reactions which we end up examining. When it happens everything changes, and even if for a magic instant, we feel "alive" and masters of our own Self; without any pressure of preoccupation we feel as if we are "in another world, in the small room of another time, another universe another deep intimacy."[1]

In writing this introduction, I intend to invite you, the reader, to take into consideration above all the immediate, surprising reaction which grabs you when you are before a work of art, when the images of a beloved film, or a famous statue, or the spectacle of a natural phenomenon bring to light in us an emotion which can open up the way for change.

From a certain perspective, art, in its varied expressions, plus cinema – my preferred choice thanks to its iconic characteristics which are so close to the oneiric dimension – is the best-fitting medium for observing these moments, thanks both to their characteristic of identification and separation, and to that of involving an encounter.

I consider the two aspects of encounter/enchantment before the beauty of the object or of loss (Investment always brings with it acceptance of the risk of loss – even traumatic loss – of the object.), to be experiences which alternate and coexist in subjective experience, laying themselves out on a continuum which runs along all of human existence. We can imagine going from the feared horror of "the object's fading" which does not survive the subject's destructivity (*Melancholia*) to the perverse outcome (*Hable con Ella* [Talk to Her]), where an act at the limit of the thinkable can contain unexpected potential for life. Meanwhile, in a different sort of complexity (*El secreto de sus ojos* [The Secret of Their Eyes]), the grief process follows a path which is already familiar with the traumatic loss of the object, known in its full beauty (a young bride raped and killed). That loss can be an inconsolable pain which will rest unchanged and lead to the victim's being banned from the human consortium as well as to the murderer's choice of revenge. It can also be unconscious transformation which leads to getting a blocked healing process back in motion (*My Architect*).

Chapter 1, "Why do we write? Psychoanalytic writing and fiction" and Chapter 2, "On the idea of beauty: standing before the Venus de Milo" could seem anomalous and out of place, inserted as they are in a collection of essays dedicated to films. However, I think of them as two key essays for understanding the choice the book is based on. The first essay deals with the topic of the written word, while the second touches on the theme of aesthetic pleasure of the object. It is always sought after as a whole, intact object whose range we can appreciate only in so far as we are able to relate to it and to tolerate its beauty in a dimension of human imperfection.

Psychoanalysis was born and remains the "talking cure," treatment through the spoken and written word, which can describe and guide towards a dimension of deeper understanding, of awareness of the complexity of one's own psychic functioning and that of others. The "word," when found/found again in its emotional fullness in art and in the analytic process, is the key element of the analytic discipline: clinically, theoretically, and when used in extension to the broader fields of culture and art.

It is necessary that we not limit our attention to pathological damage to life, and that it is with open eyes that we look at social needs, at the inherent value of trying to study and improve the quality of human life. Art can do much in this direction, in the face of deep changes brought about by new technologies in our daily life and in our way of functioning psychically and mentally. These new technologies have led to innovation and transformation which proceed at an increasing and continuous speed, so much so that our mind does not seem able to adapt at a similar rate. Virtual reality and the internet have invaded our lives in a shocking way which is still difficult to decipher, as the film *Her* demonstrates.

In collecting my papers in this book, I have chosen to leave clinical work in a strict sense, to move into the so-called "applied psychoanalysis" field. In my opinion, this is a reductive term which has, in the past, been devalued.[2] That is why I prefer to talk about bringing psychoanalytic exploration into the vast field of culture, thanks to the importance I attribute to psychoanalytic research also done outside of the setting as strictly defined, extending it in just the way Freud thought was so essential, and how he himself did, into culture in the broad sense.

In the last two decades we have moved away from the enthusiasm and security which allowed Freud, when talking about non-medical applications, to affirm,

> the assessment of psychoanalysis would be incomplete were one to leave out that, unique among medical disciplines, it has established wide ranging connections with the science of the soul and is on the verge of acquiring significance for the history of religions and civilizations, for mythology and literature, analogous to that it has for psychiatry.
>
> (Freud, 1922, p. 456)

At the time, Freud could have counted on great interest in psychoanalysis on the part of the world of culture, the humanities, and even the hard sciences, for the novelty and fascination its breakthrough discovery elicited. We contemporary analysts, on the other hand, are engaged in the struggle to win back attention from the world of culture to our discipline.

Even if psychoanalysis has its ups and downs, and this era of ours seems prey to triumphant irrationalism, psychoanalysis is and remains the most valid, broad-spectrum model for reading and interpreting the internal and external world. It is a looking-glass equipped with a lens which lets you foresee and make out hidden, concealed truths which do not have one single interpretive key.

Two essays which complete this collection are left out of the description offered above: "A brief incursion in the theatre: *Freud, or the Interpreter of Dreams*," which was inspired by having been able to enjoy, along with a dense crowd, the modernity of Freud's texts, and "A tribute to Bernardo Bertolucci," which is an acknowledgement of the director's great films and a grateful farewell on the occasion of his recent passing.

Notes

1 "When the crazy pressure of preoccupation simply vanished, and I felt myself in another world, in the small room of another time, another universe another deep intimacy. Everything changed" (Warren Poland, 2018).

2 The gigantic volume edited by Salman Aktar and Stuart Twemlow (2018), *Textbook of Applied Psychoanalysis*, with contributions by 44 authors, represents an enormous effort to de-penalize applied psychoanalysis, finally giving it its deserved recognition.

References

Aktar, Salman and Stuart Twemlow (eds), 2018. *Textbook of Applied Psychoanalysis.* London and New York: Routledge.

Freud, Sigmund. 1922. "Psycho-Analysis," and "The Libido Theory". *Standard Edition, Vol. 18.* London: Hogarth Press, p. 235.

Keats, John. 2017. *Poesie. Testo inglese a fronte.* Milan: Mondadori.

Kezich, Tullio. 2007. *Federico. Fellini, la vita e i film.* Milan: Feltrinelli.

Magherini, Graziella. 2007. *Mi Sono Innamorato di una Statua.* Florence: Nicomp L.E.

Meltzer, Donald. 1988. *The Apprehension of Beauty.* London: Karnac.

Ogden, Thomas H. 1989. *The Primitive Edge of Experience.* London: Jason Aronson Inc.

Winnicott, Donald W. 1971. "Mirror Role of Mother and Family in Child Development." In *Playing and Reality.* London: Tavistock Publications.

Chapter 1

Why do we write? Psychoanalytic writing and fiction

> Everyone who works in the domain of fiction is a bit crazy. The problem is to render this craziness interesting.
>
> François Truffaut

The remains of the analyst's day

When, as a secondary school student, I happened to read Freud's Clinical Case Studies and his prefatory letter to *A Young Girl's Diary*, I had the feeling that I had discovered something quite new, in which the beauty of writing was associated with the search for some hidden truth. In Dora, in Little Hans, and in the Wolf Man, I was able to recognize characters that I could identify with, thus discovering a new, fulfilling intimacy with myself.

Many years later, I learned that the analytic experience is based on the analyst's deep contact with herself and with her patients. This lays the foundations for the affective – somewhat paradoxical – intimacy which is the core of what the analytic dyad aims at establishing. This, however, is difficult to share with someone who has not had direct experience of it; in a way, it cannot even be said, or conveyed, lest that kind of intimacy itself might be betrayed, or deprived of its richness.

In the professional life of every analyst there are stories that transform themselves in a joyously unpredictable manner in the process of treatment, and there are others that do not change in an equally profound manner, and which we would have liked to conclude in a different way. And in the background, always present, looms one's own history, with its conflictual remains. Its fundamental features are rewritten by the analyst every time she works with her patients, revisiting her passion for psychoanalysis, and with it, also the wish to start with every new patient that complex journey which has all the characteristics of a sentimental, exploratory journey, protected by the *garde-fou* of theory (Masciangelo, 1980) and setting, but which is, nevertheless, always a self-analytic journey, a re-encounter with one's own intimacy, with one's own most hidden Self and with the other one we reflect ourselves in.

Self-analysis is self-unveiling, until we find ourselves facing some sort of incomplete sense, and then we must once again start searching, each time finding ourselves facing some sort of otherness, something or someone other from us that questions us and demands that we reinvent a language in order to continue to communicate.

All this happens in the depth of the human heart, the place of greatest intimacy; it is a place that is difficult to reach and in which it is beautiful to linger, but at the same time it is a place that eludes us, or from which we want to escape to somewhere else. It is what we call the unconscious (Schmidt-Hellerau, 2018).

Writing fiction is, in a sense, the (often exhausting) processing of an intimate encounter between what is known and what is still hidden and unknown. The same thing happens in analysis: we do not know where we are going and yet we move on, being frightened, frustrated, gratified, sometimes losing sight of the person whose story we are constructing, or rather co-constructing, in the analytic field, in a sort of reverie or countertransference phantasy.

One writes, perhaps, first and foremost for oneself, to narrate a part of one's own history which continues to appear incomplete. The hints from which we move on sometimes come from the patient, they are what I call the remains of the analytic working day.

We come across stories that seem to emerge from the dark depth of our mind, the dwelling place of creatures that take on strange and composite shapes, just like the habitat that surrounds them and in which they move. It would be easy and hasty to relegate to a dream dimension all those creatures and memories that seem unable to find shelter even in dreams. For this, it is necessary to camouflage them in the form of a "tale", with that kind of emotion that may be a shiver of fear, anxiety or passion which is associated with the "uncanny" (Freud, 1919) and which at the same time allows us to approach it, giving it a narrative form, in order to represent what comes out from the shapeless matter of which the unconscious is made; something that still has not taken – and sometimes will never take – a more comprehensible and reassuring form. There is a dimension of the uncanny, however, that does not limit itself to the Freudian definition, which has to do with the inextinguishable "nostalgia" of a state that precedes language, the ability to symbolize, the separateness, that the two unconscious subjects, analyst and analysand go through in the course of treatment.

These seem to be the surviving remains of dream reality or of a wakeful state – reveries – which emerge from the encounter with the dark depth of other minds met in the therapy room: they are the "original ingredients" in search of a shape, or simply of something in which to be placed, so as not to keep obstructing the analyst's mind.

Sometimes they describe the search for an isolated, lost Self, or they feature an object or a place capable of gathering in itself a memory, either denied or experienced – which goes beyond the subject and embraces other generations, other existences; or it is a gesture that accompanies a whole lifetime, conveying its depth. The analyst's negative capability allows her to accompany the patient in her search for those modes of expression that allow her experiences to be uttered, until they can be turned into narrations or narratives.

Thomas Ogden (2016b) writes that the conjugation of the experience of the present and the knowledge of the past in the articulation of psychoanalytic speech and clinical experience is the goal of analytic writing itself. It is, however, in the sustaining of a vital conversation or dialogue between the analytic experience and the life of the story that has been written that the art of writing psychoanalysis lies, because personal history and analytic history are intertwined in the clinical account or narrative. So what is the point of writing fiction, as Ogden himself does in his two novels: *The Part Left Out* (2013) and *The Hands of Gravity and Chance*? (2016a) Should we then think that in the clinical report that she has written, the analyst has completed her search for meaning as regards the analytic couple, her own internal truth and herself?

One is reminded of Umberto Eco (1975) when he said that what cannot be theorized about must be narrated. Could it be that this wish to write about something else on the part of the analyst is just a trivial sin of pride and omnipotence? Or could it be, instead, a search for other possible constructions and narrations that might provide an answer/interpretation which can never be completely saturated, since memories and recollections are enriched and reflected in the psychic dynamics and in Freud's notion of deferred action/*Nachträglichkeit*?

The human being is persecuted by his own mind and thoughts (Vallino, 1996), pursued by a feeling of fear which is not only linked to what has been repressed, but also to the fact that one is perhaps never sufficiently provided to face one's own emotional experiences. The need to transform fear itself fosters the need to narrate, to find words; it becomes a primordial, pulsional drive in oneself and in the Other, which prompts in the analyst the search for a way out, a possibility for growth, development, order, tranquillity and beauty.

A great writer like Elias Canetti (2017) identifies in the fear of death, that is, in something that comes before repression, the necessity to go on writing. One narrates, in his view, in order to transform fear itself, to push away the extreme limit of human existence. The writer, therefore, reacts to the mourning of the original separation (from the maternal body) with the incessant motivation to create new representational forms, each time repeating the illusion of getting closer to the perfection represented by that original, lost union.

The basic creativity of the psyche does not stop; creativity is experienced as an obscure push, which is difficult to decipher. Once the original union is lost, psychic life is structured and restructured incessantly, through a relentless creative process which can occasionally become a necessity, that is, to go on writing and thinking, as if there were only two possibilities: to be creative and give shape to new ways, or to be immobilized in psychic death. We write in order not to yield to psychic death, to keep our infantile desire alive, activating, through writing and artistic expressions, those resistances, defences, censures and transformations which allow for the knowledge of one's internal world, in a sort of oscillation between approaching and distancing ourselves from the abyss of unknowable experiences which we constantly struggle to represent. The need to write, in this perspective, is linked to one's incessant internal dynamism and therefore to the process of working through mourning.

Whoever writes, whether she is an analyst or not, must be able to find a "technical/creative" language which can be shared, which can express her subjectivity, but also in order for others to follow a pathway similar to hers. Her goal is to provide shapes and meanings which can help to express what is striking in its intensity but keeps avoiding – in its entirety – any representation and thinkability.

This is what Freud had realized when he turned art in general – and writing in particular – into a precious ally for disclosing the truth of psychic mechanisms. Probably following an opposite pathway, the contemporary writer Annie Ernaux (2016) asks herself in her latest novel: "What's the point of writing … if not to dig up things, maybe just one thing, irreducible to any sort of explanation … one thing … that can help us to understand – to tolerate – what is happening and what we are doing?" When we write fiction are we perhaps pursuing the enigma of an intimacy with ourselves and the Other, whether they are patients or readers, of the kind of encounter about which Freud wrote in 1905, "Every finding of an object is in fact a re-finding of it."?

Not everything that emerges from the encounter between two unconscious minds in the analytic room can be shared, because of the unacknowledged limits of the analyst, her "blind spots" (Guignard, 1996), or because of the new dimension of contemporary analysis, which has extended its boundaries to new pathologies and has changed the notion of interpretation, which now tends to be unsaturated, thus opening up, (ad infinitum?) the possibility of finding new meanings, interpretations, and narrations.

A clinical vignette

As an example of what I said before, I end with a short story about a memory that slowly acquires meaning and shape, re-emerging in the analyst with intense emotion: something which happened in the past and that returns as a mental state which silently finds its way during a session and which helps the patient remember; however, it does not end there: instead, it reawakens in the analyst too, the memory of an event experienced in the past but not fully thought about. The story describes that ineffable instant in which the need to endure waiting leaves the dimension of frustrating negative capability and reaches an area of suspension, the prelude to remembrance, which is retrieved and savoured in all its evocative fullness since it is no longer isolated by affect (Green, 1978).

The memory that emerges in the story is charged with nostalgia, but the ability to mourn what has been lost and has trapped the mind in an idealized dimension can finally become the prelude for a transformation. Now it is no longer laden with loss, but indeed enriched by nostalgia, that is "longing and loss." It can be read as an attempt to capture that particular experience of suspense, excitement and apprehension that lies between the desire to prolong the prelude of things and the return to everyday reality; everything is then magnified by the uniqueness and the enormity of the expected event in that morning of the past. There is something that becomes an enormous metaphor, just as feelings experienced in adolescence can be, with the expectation of a life shared in the resonance of a group of peers, "those young boys, companions of her fairer season" (Leopardi, 1825).

There is an expectation for a surprising awakening, in a moment which is halfway between "an air which is no longer wintry and is still not spring-like," it is the moment of imminent change, or of insight, an oscillation between something extraordinary and the anxiety of something terrible that might happen; something that in any case will be unique and irreplicable. And then comes the relief of not having lost the normality of daily life and the slight regret of having already experienced the unforgettable moment.

The description of the past event is activated in the analyst by the atmosphere of a session in which the memories of the patient, which had been blocked by repetition for a long time, can re-emerge. On that day, the patient had entered the therapy room carrying with her the physical sensation of an undefinable "air;" in that moment, however, instead of complaining – as many other times in the past – about the town's impossible climate, or her oncoming cold, she was left suspended in a different sort of nostalgia which was heralding something new. After her initial irritation at the thought that the session would follow the same sterile pathway, the analyst had perceived the patient's wish to share with her "that air" and to understand what it might signify. As the session progressed, the analytic couple were committed to finding the words to describe the intense feeling, charged with emotions and affects, which had been roused by the physical sensation, until the analyst said "an air that feels like the end of winter and the beginning of spring: the kind of air that anticipates changes." It was one of those moments in which the analyst while interpreting, put into words what the patient was ready to understand (Busch, 2014). At that point, the patient was able to recall memories of her adolescence, retrieving her past desires, dreams and disappointments, but above all a kind of vital energy that for a long time she had experienced as being extinguished and harnessed.

On leaving the office, the analyst, still immersed in her patient's words, was struck by a gust of that same air and gave in to her own chain of associations, retrieving the nuances of a memory of her own, of an event from her past which she had experienced, but not thought about. She could have let it fall into a dimension or dark space of her mind, but she felt that it had the power of that unforgettable season in life, which is adolescence.

I have tried to depict a mental space that silently finds its way, that the analyst perceives, starting from a physical experience, which activates memory and allows for the powerful re-emergence of that very moment. The analyst/narrator is captured by it, and she lapses into a chain of associations, retrieving the nuances of that memory, of that event, which could not be thought in all its complexity because it was too charged with emotion and excitement. Silently and surprisingly, that feeling is renewed, in all its power, in the here and now of the analyst, prolonged after the session.

Sometimes a memory like this takes years to emerge, through flashes or stubborn lapses of memory, and momentary revelations that are enriching, but still not sufficient. And only at the end can they be seen as part of the complex and tormented interweaving of human affects, finally finding a way to be revealed by means of the outline of a narration, so as to retrieve a fuller meaning and ultimately discard what has not been completely detoxified before.

The analyst/narrator experiences in herself the moment of bewilderment, of puzzlement before of a natural event that fosters a sort of "oceanic" feeling, something in front of which, "for a while my heart is lost in fear" as Giacomo Leopardi wrote in his poem "Infinity."

Mardi Gras – Ash Wednesday

As soon as she left her office, she was surprised by the crisp, icy-cold air and the clear light of a late winter evening. She remembered that it was Mardi Gras: a sad carnival of crisis and unemployment, but the kids were laughing and joking as always, throwing foam and talcum powder at one another.

For a long time, she had not paid attention to that, but in the past few years every Mardi Gras reminded her of a particular one, of many years before.

She had gone to a small party at somebody's place, who knows who: she remembered that she had felt rather cold in her little black dress, with short sleeves and a chaste boat neck.

The party was simple, without masks, as they were not common in those years.

She drank some sweet, sparkling wine, laughed at the jokes and did some rock 'n' roll and ballroom dancing, letting all the occasional suitors irritate her cheek with their badly shaved or poorly trimmed beards, without being able to avoid feeling that something was missing. It was probably, for her, one of those intermediate moments between one crush and another, a prelude, charged with expectations, between freedom and loneliness.

She came home late, everyone was already sleeping; the following morning – she had forgotten about it – her secondary school class was supposed to go to the hillside to see the sun's total eclipse, a momentous event for which their physics teacher had been preparing them for months.

She was probably sleeping deeply when she woke up with a start, feeling that she had gone to sleep only a moment before, and she remembered about the trip all of a sudden, fearing that the coach would leave without her, and that all her classmates would already be ready and waiting in front of the school. She dressed up quickly and ran, ran until she felt sick, and she managed to join the group just they were about to leave. She was the last one to get on the coach, among her mates' joking remarks and their usual quips. Then everyone started shouting, as the coach took the uphill road in the crisp morning air. It was an incredibly crystal-clear morning; the air was no longer wintry, but not yet spring-like.

Once they reached their destination, they all got off the coach, screaming and joking, and they headed for the location chosen by their teacher, who was guiding them, pompous, and conscious of the "keynote lecture" that he was about to give to his students.

They put on their sunglasses, following his instructions. She had found a very old pair at home and had put them in her pocket at the very last moment, without knowing whose they were. It should be said that sunglasses were an unusual item in those days, something that very few people wore, and generally only in the mountains or at the coast.

The darkness fell all of a sudden.

Close to her feet she saw a blooming crocus closing again; she saw animals suddenly cringing; she saw quick hands closing the shutters of a farmstead, afraid of God's judgement. Then, in a moment, all was dark and silent.

Even they, the students, were silenced by the spectacle, and they waited, holding their breath shivering with fear, for the sun to come out again. And it did. Once again, the sun granted its splendid encore: the crocus opened up again, the rooster crowed for a second time, the peasants reopened their windows and doors, and the students clapped their hands, relieved, making fun of themselves and of their stupid fears.

She wondered yet again what had made that day so special, which ingredients had blended together in her memory in such an indelible manner. The only total solar eclipse of the twentieth century, a class of secondary school students on a field trip, a hilly landscape, a wonderful winter dawn, two mismatched adults (the driver and the physics teacher), a 1960s coach, of a faded blue colour, which slightly veered when it went uphill?

Indeed, everything had blended together in a surprising amalgamation of vital drives, yet confused, fed by the hormonal storm of twenty teenage students on a field trip, with their baggage of new and old loves, loyalty and betrayal, jealousy and envy, fantasized and illicit sex, secrets and lies, expectations and disappointments, anxieties, fears, and so on and so forth. An almost incalculable sum of narcissisms, each one of which had seen something about itself in the unique spectacle of the sun that eclipsed and then rose again. In a moment of awe before the wonderful show of "mother nature", everyone had been able to perceive what would happen in the immediate future: the possibility of triumphing, the anxiety of being eclipsed, and the uncertainty of getting a second chance.

And one could also mention the narcissism of the physics teacher who – apart from the fact that, for once, he would not have to struggle to get attention and silence from his class – had already foretasted his triumph over those students who loved literature and philosophy more than his own subject, and over his colleagues, none of whom, indeed, had such an ace up their sleeves!

All this came alive again to her, that morning, in the crystal-clear, icy-cold air of an Ash Wednesday many years later; an ordinary day when the sun would not rise a second time. But she could always hope that she might be given yet another small chance.

Conclusions

Among the qualities that a writer must possess, there is an ability to find a technical, creative language that she can share with her audience; and through the expression of her own subjectivity she must also allow other people to follow pathways which can be different or similar to her own, but which must be equally capable of leading to emotions that can be represented.

The analyst must do something similar in order to allow her interpretation or reconstruction to be shared by the patient. In this sense, both art and psychoanalysis dare to seek an expression for what used to seem uncanny, ineffable and unspeakable, and they construct a language of words, sounds, colours and shapes – also enriched with rediscovered affects – which is finally adequate for expressing what had eluded any previous definition. Freudianly, we might say that art is a precious ally in the struggle to assert the truth of certain psychic constructs and mechanisms. Together, following different pathways, psychoanalytic writing and fiction provide a binocular vision that focuses on the same object, allowing for the mutual realisation of the perceived object as well as of the subject.

References

Busch, Fred. 2014. *Creating a Psychoanalytic Mind: A Psychoanalytic Method and Theory.* London and New York: Routledge.

Canetti, Elias. 2017. *Il Libro contro la Morte.* Milan: Adelphi Edizioni.

Eco, Umberto. 1975. *Trattato di Semiotica Generale.* Milan: Feltrinelli.

Ernaux, Annie. 2016. *Memoire de fille.* Paris: Gallimard.

Freud, Sigmund. 1905. "Three Essays on the Theory of Sexuality", *Standard Edition, Vol. 7.* London: Hogarth Press, p. 125.

Freud, Sigmund. 1919. "The Uncanny", *Standard Edition, Vol. 17*. London: Hogarth Press, p. 219.

Green, André. 1978. *Il Discorso Vivente*. Milan: Raffaello Cortina Editore.

Guignard, Florence. 1996. *Au vif de l'infantile: aujourd'hui. Reflections sur la situation analytique*. Paris: Éditions d'Itaque.

Leopardi, Giacomo. 1994. "The Village Saturday" (p. 106), "The Infinite" (p. 53). In *I Canti*. Manchester: Carcanet Press.

Masciangelo, Pier Mario. 1980. "Assetti, funzionamenti e relazioni perverse. Metapsicologia di un'esperienza clinica." In A.A. Semi (ed.), *Trattato di Psicoanalisi*. Milan: Raffaello Cortina Editore.

Ogden, Thomas. 2013. *The Parts Left Out*. London: Karnac.

Ogden, Thomas. 2016a. *The Hands of Gravity and Chance*. London: Karnac.

Ogden, Thomas. 2016b. *Reclaiming Unlived Lives: Experiences in Psychoanalysis*. London and New York: Routledge.

Schmidt-Hellerau, Cordelia. 2018. "The intimacy of the analyst writing fiction." *Driven to Survive*. New York: International Psychoanalytic Books, pp. 445–452.

Vallino, Dina. 1996. "Postfazione." In Antonino Ferro, *Nella stanza d'analisi*. Milan: Raffaello Cortina Editore, pp. 157–163.

Chapter 2

On the idea of beauty

Standing before the Venus de Milo

> In praise of imperfection which does not make us homogeneous. Rather, it makes us different and unique.
>
> Anonymous

The vision of the world sculpted by Classical and Hellenistic Greek artists at the peak of their splendour seems to have disappeared forever. That very vision, which embodies our ideal of classical perfection and human body harmony, is reflected – among others – by the Venus de Milo, an ancient Greek statue I would like to discuss here.

From the beginning of the twentieth century onwards, art has gone very much beyond limits: the perception of the real world, of the human form, of the natural and metropolitan landscape having disappeared, it is almost as if artists had been forced to try and attain a limit which might embody the ability of the Self to survive, in spite of its being more and more under pressure, while being endowed with ever more refined senses which can apprehend the molecular essence of the object itself, its eyes expecting to see the infinitesimally small, its ears wanting to hear inaudible sounds.

As Adela Abella (2012) keenly highlights, some contemporary artists seem to be dissecting fragments of matter so as to show their aesthetic potential in the field of music and the visual arts. At the same time, works of art are being assembled and installed which – over and above the special meaning conferred by the authors – remind us of the effort to reproduce and to show the very special kind of creature humans have actually become: unfortunately, this new creature sometimes looks like a poorly drawn and badly assembled Frankenstein dominated by the death drive rather than impelled by the life drive.

The boundaries of what can be perceived and thought – although progressively moving forward thanks to ever more extensive research – always end up facing a limit, whereas art, by nature, flourishes at the threshold of what is inexpressibly mysterious, where an eternal play finds its beginning whereby the world is recreated, inscribed, or else painted over and over again, its sounds and colours endlessly reproduced and changed.

Contemporary humans know that their environment is threatened by resource depletion and overpopulation. They constantly receive almost real-time updates of what is happening in every corner of the world and are bombarded with visual stimuli and overwhelming amounts of information. Advertising and media help them develop a refined aesthetic sense, yet they seem to be in need of art more than ever. But what do they look for when they look at art and what do they find in it?

Ancient art seems to quench man's thirst for a lost world which appears all the more beautiful as we are now running the risk of destroying it forever: a world we can now only dream of, which produced works of art commissioned by a privileged, ruling class who knew how to keep the horrors of war, famine and the darkest despair completely separate from the pomp and splendour they could surround themselves with.

Contemporary art, however, is often provocative, irritating: it can make you feel ill at ease, it can be startling and amazing. Beauty and its reproduction – for centuries the basic criteria of any artwork – are now almost felt to be a hindrance to artistic research. Rather than hinting at what is lost, contemporary artists seem to be striving for meaning in contemporary world chaos, trying to help us think about our anxieties and sorrows, about present-time traumatic events without offering any answer – they do not have any answers – but rather, raising new questions, the way Bion would do.

For instance, let us consider Anselm Kiefer, a distinguished, contemporary German painter and sculptor. His works of art exert a fascinating and disquieting power on us. Mixing materials such as sand, sunflower seeds, lead, dried flower stems, he evokes images of the Shoah, ashes, winds of war, ferocious dictatorships, and falling stars. He offers a terrible and sublime mixture of nature and culture while encompassing the beauty and aberration of both, so as to make us understand what we material twentieth-century humans are made of, those who survived the horrors of the so-called "short century", their flesh wounded by what cannot even be contemplated. In the analysts' rooms, this unthinkable sorrow emerges from transgenerational memories: during the slow, tenacious analytic work a patient's memory denies, deletes, but also reconstructs and constructs over and over again.

Kiefer maintains that art has a transcendent and disquieting function: it cannot escape the past nor can it elude the future. It is the motionless universe scrutinizing its own progression, it is man affirming the uniqueness of his presence and expecting from the artist that the creator/creature be redeemed: globally, it is a deep sense of sacrifice which the artist must make on our behalf. Contemporary art in particular hints at our fragmented, split and chaotic parts while stimulating a wish for integration and restructuring of those very elements which art itself proved to be destructured.

Why, then, does the Venus de Milo – with her enchanting, very classical forms – still exert such a powerful fascination over the public as they pass her at the Louvre Museum, so much so that she has become the most popular artwork in the Western world? Every year, six and a half million out of eight million people visiting the Louvre stand before this statue and contemplate its beauty. What do twenty-first century men and women see in her? Are we allowed to think that this art object has become a sort of fetish, or else this disparaging explanation – betraying a derogatory, intellectual attitude towards the masses – simply relieves us from the need to look for a different explanation?

While I am sure you are all acquainted with the history of this statue, I would like to offer you a few historical facts. The Venus de Milo is a 202 cm-high, Parian marble statue. A Hellenistic work dated to around 130 BCE; its composition is a mixture of earlier styles from the Classical period. Originally, its beauty led experts to mistakenly believe it to be an original work by Praxiteles dating to the Golden Age of Classicism (4th century, BCE): however, following a thorough analysis of the technique employed to sculpt it, it was then attributed to Alexandros of Antioch (1st century BCE).

The history of its recovery is fascinating and romantic, as befits a real beauty: in 1820, while ploughing his fields, the peasant Yorgos Kentrotas discovered two large, broken pieces of a marble statue on the Greek island of Milos, at that time under Ottoman rule. Having overcome his initial astonishment at the find, he hid the statue with the help of some relatives all the while thinking that he might as well earn some money by selling it. An initial and fractious dispute of possession of the statue was finally resolved by its purchase as a gift to Louis XVIII. A year later, King Louis XVIII donated the statue to the Louvre and on 24 May it was put on public display. The event was garnered great attention by the French: five years earlier, France had returned the Venus de'Medici to Italy after it had been "acquired" by Napoleon Bonaparte. Now they wanted to secure a new Venus for themselves, even more beautiful than the first one!

A fresh dispute – among "brothers", we might say – arose concerning its restoration: did the statue hold an apple in its left hand or not? Did it rest on a pillar or not? Would it have to be restored or should it remain in the state it had been found? In the end, the wise decision was taken not to restore it: however, in order to soothe the spirits, the honour of the final decision was bestowed on the King,[1] who was called on to perform his paternal function we might say! When confronted with such feminine beauty, how could we possibly blame those who first discovered the Venus, or the experts arguing over whether to restore it or not, and indeed, they continued to debate this question for over ten years, that is, up until 1833. In fact, apart from one famous detractor, Pierre Auguste Renoir, who admiring a different type of woman, called it the "big gendarme", the Venus de Milo is considered the most classical representation of feminine beauty.

During the twentieth century, as was the case with many antiquities, they became idealized objects; even the breathtakingly beautiful Venus de Milo was paid homage on the one hand while becoming an object of ridicule on the other.

I am thinking of the way its image is used for advertising purposes, but also of the wonderful appearance of Isabelle, the main character in Bernardo Bertolucci's *The Dreamers* (2003), dressed as the Venus de Milo without arms,[2] or else of its disquieting version in *Boxing Helena* (1993) by film director Jennifer Chambers Lynch. In this movie, a surgeon amputates the legs and arms of the unfortunate woman with whom he is infatuated, without having his feelings returned.

Apart from being astonished by the Venus's degree of fame and admiration, probably by now you will be rightfully wondering why on earth it came to my mind to talk about this statue.

At this point I think I should explain that my thoughts on this statue and on the great fascination it still evokes nowadays were stirred by a piece written by Umberto Eco (2012), the Italian semiologist, where he states that the Venus de Milo enchants its viewers despite its missing arms, or rather, *precisely thanks to its missing arms.* This very statement – in fact quite surprising – that the Venus enchants its viewers "precisely thanks to its missing arms" made me pause and reflect on his words.

It is certainly true that, while contemplating the Venus, we are inevitably captured by the wish to imagine the "everything" that is lost forever while indulging in a sweet melancholy evoked by the thought of human transience and the transience of beauty in particular. These feelings are intertwined and inevitably tied to the idea of destiny of all things, as Freud wrote in the opening sentences of his wonderful essay "On Transience", published in 1915.

> Not long ago I went on a summer walk through a smiling countryside in the company of a taciturn friend and of a young but already famous poet. The poet admired the beauty of the scene around us but felt no joy in it. He was disturbed by the thought that all this beauty was fated to extinction, that it would vanish when winter came, like all human beauty and all the beauty and splendour that men have created or may create. All that he would otherwise have loved and admired seemed to him to be shorn of its worth by the transience which was its doom.
>
> (Freud, 1915, p. 173, translation by James Strachey)

In this essay Freud reminds us that in order to get pleasure from all that is beautiful, it is necessary to tolerate its loss and the "psychic rebellion" against it (ibid., p. 174). This is the only chance we have if we want to regain possession of the conflicting affects through which we feel tied to the lost love-object, that is, to all that we would have loved and admired but which appears "shorn of its worth by the transience which (was) is its doom" (ibid., p. 173).

Longing is a terrible feeling as are the feelings commonly associated with loss, but both may foster the seeds of creativity defying death and mourning,[3] trying to re-create and repair the Self in search of the image of what has been traumatically lost. The temptation to deny loss and the passing of time and to re-create the object exactly as it was before trauma is always very strong. For instance, let us think about the raging debate over how to reconstruct La Fenice in Venice following its destruction by fire, or many other great monuments which had been damaged following war, bombardment, or natural disasters (Goretti, 1997). The core of those debates was whether to reconstruct them exactly as they had been before the destruction, as if to deny what had happened.

It is all the more surprising that nothing of the kind ever concerned the Venus de Milo, which seems to be loved specifically because it shows the damage due to the passing of time.

We certainly admire her formal beauty, and the lost world from which she originates; a world which lies within each of us and whose loss we mourn. All this does not simply refer to the outer world – the historical past – but it also concerns our inner dimension: the perfect incompleteness of the statue exerts a powerful fascination on the latter, because it makes it possible to get closer to the beauty of the object, as is the case at the origin of mental life, when the aesthetic/ecstatic object is the mother's breast. Meltzer (1988) derived from Bion the concept of "aesthetic conflict" reflecting the infant's conflict between attraction towards the dazzling beauty of the breast and the maternal face and the panic and terror of what is hidden in its inner reality: the premonition of abandonment, of the absence of the object, of the anguish arising from the difficulty to tolerate frustration and the destructive rage that may follow.

In contemporary art, we have learned to love imperfections and the unfinished almost more than that which is entirely completed, to love sketches more than drawings, as if we find it challenging to feel mirrored by intact, perfect forms – as was the case in the past – as if we needed things which have only been drafted, unsaturated, imperfect things to reassure us because we feel better suited to a world whose imperfections are so familiar.

To put it simply, that which is imperfect is less enviable for us, as people of the 3rd millenia, less distant from us and so we prefer it and find it comforting knowing that time goes by inexorably, that we are no longer at the dawn of history but rather, that a two-millennia period of history is already behind us. What happened during the twentieth century in particular has robbed us forever of our innocence.

Umberto Eco clearly demonstrates profound, refined knowledge of the human spirit, particularly in its exclusively human characteristic – narcissism. Being an attentive art expert, that is, being a "connoisseur" of one of the highest expressions of humanity, Eco captures the "healthy" narcissism of the museum visitor who loves art and finds enjoyment in it; he appreciates the unconscious pang inevitably experienced by the viewer when standing before the genius and bravura of others, contemporaries, or predecessors as they may be. As Nietzsche rightly pointed out, whenever we stand before a work of art, for a very short instant we feel we share the artist's brilliance: we belong to one and the same humanity, and the beauty of any work of art helps us feel less anonymous and powerless, helping us retrieve a small part of our unrepeatable uniqueness in a world which is ever more anonymous and overcrowded, where it is easier to feel lost and forgotten rather than feel we are an acknowledged part of one and the same community.

Spellbound by the mastery of the artist who sculpted the Venus de Milo, the viewer should find comfort in the thought that a human like himself could conceive such perfect beauty. And who would have dared try to measure up to such perfection, setting about reshaping Venus's arms as beautiful as the originals must have been, with the right arm poised in front of her chest so as to hold up the drapery around her midriff and with the left arm thrust up and forwards with an apple in hand, the gift of Paris for her, Venus, the one he had chosen as the most beautiful of all goddesses? Comfort also seems to derive from the very amputation of both arms caused by fate, as if it were the price spectators had to pay to their feelings of ambivalence and envy when standing before perfection. Nothing more human than that, after all.

In discussing the theme of the apprehension of beauty, Donald Meltzer (1988) – whom I have already quoted – states that we are not moved by the beauty of the object, but instead by its transience. He describes the "aesthetic conflict" facing the newborn when he is exposed to the splendour of the maternal breast and face, that is, in the presence of the object he foresees its absence and ensuing pain: the object cannot be fully owned, its absolute beauty will remain inaccessible, unsustainable. It is only possible to obtain pleasure from it for a short while, provided that the need to get hold of it and consume it does not grow so strong as to lead to its destruction. When that does happen, the disappearance of the attacked object causes a paralyzing feeling of persecution which – among others – makes real aesthetic enjoyment impossible.

In Bion's terms, as revisited by Civitarese "we are moved by the 'no-breast' or, to be more precise, by the 'no-thing'" (Civitarese, 2011, p. 115), that is, we are enchanted with the temporary perception of the absence of the object from which thought can emerge. Contemplating an aesthetic object and experiencing pleasure from its beauty is only possible after mourning the ephemeral nature of human life and all things, after having developed the ability to feel confident that it will reappear. In fact, it is the very expectation that the object will appear again which promotes an experience of harmony and attunement with the object itself which is lost-found, found-created, as Winnicott would have it, allowing thought and a sense of Self to emerge. Therefore, we might say that the Venus de Milo is offering us a partial and temporary resolution of the Meltzerian "aesthetic conflict": while contemplating her beauty, for a brief moment we get closer to the Bionian "O", that is, to the absolute truth, to the unknowable which will remain unattainable but towards which we will forever strive. Umberto Eco's analysis is admirable because it captures the exciting contradiction nested in beauty and imperfection.

Moreover, we might think that the enchanted visitor, spellbound before the goddess's beauty, is taken to an area of the psyche where there are no needs, deficits or unfulfilled desires, where others have not yet appeared as well-defined figures, where the Ego can relive the state defined by Winnicott's sentence: "I am the breast", the original sense of being merged with the object, the very magic moment of infantile omnipotence (Winnicott, 1975). This may happen in an instant when, as we contemplate a work of art, we experience a touch of immortality before differentiation between Ego and the object sets in and deception ensues. For a brief moment, the viewer standing before the Venus de Milo ends up in contact with a remote, secret area of his psyche where her being is enough, where s/he has no need of arms extended toward the other so as to ask or receive.

Is this the sublime condition the sculptor reproduced, aided by fate and the passing of time, is this the very condition which leaves us in ecstatic contemplation of the perfection of a being which needs nothing else beyond oneself? For a moment, we too relive that very enjoyable state, as if we were at the origins of existence, with no other need but to contemplate – through that wondrous, yet maimed statue – our inimitable uniqueness.

So perhaps more than a problem of imperfection, we are facing the problem of seeing oneself reflected in a state of perfection: condemned to a continuous search for the other, for some moments the human being enjoys the fullness of Self and therefore needs no arms with which to ask, to seize, to demonstrate her capacity. She is a human simply affirming her existence which is incomparable, in itself imperfectly perfect, while s/he sees herself in the image of the beautiful sphinx which stands before her, the most enigmatic part of her Self and of the other being which s/he must eternally compare herself with. A poor, helpless creature when facing death, yet wonderful in her irreducible uniqueness. Each viewer can engage in dialogue with this wonderful, enigmatic, unknown woman of the past, a silent and ecstatic dialogue during which she can reveal to contemporary man the secret allowing her to resist till the present time. Perhaps this is the very secret we would like to share with her: how to endure the passing of time, entering a no-time dimension which is the time/no-time of desire, within which something of each of us survives.

The father of psychoanalysis has an ace up his sleeve which may help us decipher the mystery of the success of the Venus de Milo. During a visit to the Louvre in 1895, Freud wrote to his fiancée Martha that he had been enchanted by and had greatly admired an army of Greek and Roman statues, among which he had caught sight of and felt moved by the "famous Venus de Milo, her arms missing." His future collection would include a small bronze statue of Venus, an ageless woman, young and charming, strongly erotized like the *matrem nudam*, missing "those" arms which hold and support. A "classical" representation of Amalia as the young and irresistible mother of little Siggy,[4] the son who was destined to nourish his young, beautiful mother's narcissism? Venus missing her arms is a symbol for the eternally longed-for *matrem nudam* belonging to collective imagination, a symbol for eternal youth, for the fixation to a unique moment of fullness of the Self when no other need is felt but to keep on enjoying that very moment which is set out of time and which bears the promise of immortality and perfection, two states human beings mostly yearn for.

Conclusions

All in all, what do contemporary people see in the Venus de Milo? Do they see a long lost form of perfection, do they consider it proof of a kind of beauty we have manipulated, disassembled and reassembled to such an extent that we are no longer able to find pleasure in it if we are not further manipulating and working on it?

The goddess without arms would then stand for all that humanity has lost, sublime works which were produced at a time when beauty was a rare and precious gift, so much so that it would only be considered an attribute of goddesses or demigods. Standing before the Venus de Milo we nostalgically and regretfully reflect on the transience of all human things, on the greatness we can attain and – as I said before – on the perfection of being: for a brief moment, perfection is attained in its uniqueness, a state which fascinates us because it proves it is possible to resist, to survive and, therefore, to keep our most catastrophic anguish under control while experiencing a touch of immortality, the promise conveyed to an infant by his mother's loving look.

The aesthetic experience as such is tied to the destiny of emotions in general and to the specific ability to be moved by beauty. It gives us the chance to introject the goodness and integrity of the object or else to feel exposed to its destructive projection (Meltzer 1988[1963], p. 244). If, before a work of art, we feel touched, this experience gives us the possibility to soothe our anguish: poets were aware of it well before us, since Homer wrote that beauty is "the breast which makes us forget our anguish."[5]

On the contrary, those who cannot allow themselves to feel positive emotions – because they would be experienced as too strong and, therefore, potentially dangerous – turn the object, even an artistic one, into something inanimate, which they can only grasp the formal aspects of, making a fetish out of it. Rather than loving a work of art, they only appreciate its commercial value or else they use it for exhibitionistic purposes: I saw it too! Recently, it has become very trendy to take a selfie before La Gioconda (Mona Lisa) or the Venus de Milo!

Notes

1 Actually, the decision was taken by Antoine Quatremère de Quincy, Secretary to the Royal Academy of the Fine Arts.
2 The obtained, visual effect is, in fact, an optical illusion: the wonderful protagonist is wearing long black gloves while the scene is shot against a black background.
3 "Creativity is Eros's defiance of Thanatos" (Poland, 2014).
4 "Mein goldener Sigi" [My golden Siggy]: as Amalia liked to call her beloved, first-born child.
5 Homer. *The Iliad*, XXII.

References

Abella, Adela. 2012. "John Cage and W.R. Bion: an exercise in interdisciplinary dialogue." *International Journal of Psychoanalysis* 93(3) (June): 717–731.

Bertolucci, Bernardo. (dir.) *The Dreamers*. 2003. Rome: Medusa Distribuzione. Film.

Bion, Wilfred R. 1965. *Transformations: Changes from Learning to Growth*. New York: Basic Books.

Chambers Lynch, Jennifer. (dir.) *Boxing Helena*. 1993. Los Angeles: Orion Classics. Film.

Civitarese, Giuseppe. 2011. *La violenza delle emozioni. Bion e la psicoanalisi post-bioniana*. Milan: Raffaello Cortina.

Eco, Umberto. 2012. "Perché è così bella la Venere senza braccia: Il fascino della Venere di Milo." *La Repubblica*, 7 July.

Freud, Sigmund. 1915. "On Transience." *Standard Edition, Vol. 14*. London: Hogarth Press, p. 305.

Gay, Peter. 1988. *Freud: A Life for Our Time*. New York and London: W.W. Norton & Co.

Goretti, Giovanna. 1997. "L'incendio della Fenice e le difese collettive." *Rivista di Psicoanalisi* XLIII(1): 51–61. Rome: Borla.

Meltzer, Donald. 1988*The Apprehension of Beauty*. London: Karnac.

Poland, Warren S. 2014. *Intimacy and Separateness in Psychoanalysis*. London: Routledge.

Trapanese, Gemma. 2012. "figlia d'oro." In Patrizia Cupelloni (ed.), *Psicoanaliste*. Milan: Franco Angeli Editore, pp. 82–102.

Winnicott, Donald W. 1975. *Through Paediatrics to Psycho-Analysis: Collected Papers*. London: Karnac Classics.

Chapter 3

Traumatic states of the self

Castaway by Robert Zemeckis[1]

Through psychoanalysis, we have come to understand that cinema facilitates the representation of unconscious impressions and fears (Gabbard, 1997) and constitutes an unexpected source for exploring, at greater depths, experiences that are often beyond the intentions of filmmakers and financiers. This seems to be the case with *Castaway* (2000) by Robert Zemeckis, which, conceived as a mass-consumption film, ends up revealing the typical anxieties of contemporary man having to come to terms with his most elementary needs and recognize his affective dependence. These anxieties extend from the vision of becoming a homeless urban reject to the modern nightmare of being suddenly reduced to affective homelessness, marooned on an atoll of unreachable solitude. This may lead someone to 'shipwreck' on the analyst's couch and there begin a long and difficult voyage.

The ever-topical setting of the film is a desert island, where the individual must come face-to-face with his limitations. In the eighteenth-century world of Robinson Crusoe (Defoe, 1719), the relationship with the inner and external environment, however apparently hostile and unknown, is in the end reassuring, showing the individual's capacity to take possession of the surroundings and become enriched through contact. On the contrary, Chuck Nolan (Tom Hanks), a FedEx manager, faces the paradox of being accustomed to living in an external environment of growing comfort and ease, in contrast to his inner world, where his relationship with his objects lacks continuity and he runs the risk of losing contact with them. In the novel, the island where Crusoe was shipwrecked, although at first deserted and inhospitable, gradually fills up with animals and eventually even a human being, called Friday. This involves the reader in an exciting and enriching fantasy. However, in *Castaway*, the modern spectator feels a growing anxiety, landing together with Chuck Nolan in a 'world' where life is increasingly suspended and stationary, where the only other human being is the corpse of another unfortunate traveller.

The man we see in the opening scenes of the film is overweight and excitable; he harangues an audience of incredulous Russians whom he addresses through an interpreter and whom he exhorts to speed up things to the maximum, as required by the functioning of FedEx, his employer. This corporation is similar to the functioning of the contemporary film industry. There is no real contact between him and the world that surrounds him; the group of diffident, slightly curious Russians represents a possible interior scenario, in which he must continually exhort part of the self to keep up a complex defensive structure. Speed, the optimized use of time, travel and communication in real time (but seldom face-to-face) – these myths form the pillar of our modern world. In the film, they are carried to excess, thus preparing the viewer for impending catastrophe. Chuck Nolan's great to-do is for the sake of delivering parcels everywhere in the world as quickly as possible. It is a challenge against gravity, as well as time, to fly with winged feet like Mercury, the company trademark. To win his inner challenge against time, it seems he is ready to do anything: he is alleged to have stolen, or as he claims "borrowed", a bicycle from a disabled child. At another level, this child could be seen as an image of a harmless self, whose immobility and slowness are seen as intolerable to the adult Chuck.

The viewer begins to realize that the future castaway is an individual on the run, as if from the permanent threat of losing contact with his world and his love object. Speed and haste are also linked with the compulsion to check the reliability and continuity of the world of objects and affects that surrounds him and that he might lose at any moment. The reliability and sticking power of his relationship with this world is continually subjected to testing by a maniacal reparation, which does not achieve its intended goal, but imprisons it in compulsive repetitiveness. He is constantly sending messages to the woman he loves, but always abandons her while on business.

The catastrophe occurs during an aeroplane flight, the means of transport that most exalts the maniacal, grandiose self, but that also most reveals its fragility. The crash catapults him from his world to an atoll off navigational routes, forces him to confront his needs and throws him into a physical and psychic wild state. The scenes of the air crash are probably the greatest and most perturbing in the film, almost as if to emphasize the fascination of the trauma, both feared and denied. It stresses that survival is a matter of chance, thus flying in the face of the narcissistic preoccupation with unlimited efficiency, on which the hero has founded his security.

The sudden fall from apparent material ease and superficial affective comfort (the main character has everything one can wish for, including a mutual loving relationship) to hardship, deprivation and difficulty becomes the sign of an inner world that pushes the protagonist towards psychic wildness and isolation. There, on the atoll, his only interlocutor will be the dummy, named 'Wilson', assembled on a sudden creative intuition, which saves him from psychological collapse. Wilson constitutes his imaginary companion (cf. *The Secret Sharer*, Conrad, 1912). Onto this dummy, Chuck projects all the anger he feels towards himself and others, in order to not be destroyed. It is the mortally wounded part of the self, almost annihilated by the trauma, that must be angrily kicked to impress on it a forced movement, like that of a rolling ball. His sole remaining links with the lost affective world are the portrait of his fiancée, Kelly (Helen Hunt), inside the pocket watch she gave him, which stopped at the time of the traumatic event, and the only FedEx parcel he will not open on the atoll. Having lost the frenetic and accelerated sense of time of his previous existence, he finds himself in a timeless zone, which is revealed in his unsuccessful attempt to set up continuity with a discontinued inner object. The intermittent light on his fiancée's portrait, and his need to switch on the little flashlight in the dead of night to see her face, are symbols of a primitive dependency, in which closing one's eyes or turning off the light is the same as losing the reassuring affective presence and falling into isolation. This testifies to an affective catastrophe when he is physically separated from the object, which has caused the "wrecking" of a part of the self, and is shut up in a psychic retreat (Steiner, 1993), an internal atoll, to which the trauma pushes him back, forcing him to feel again the grief of loss in corporal, as well as psychic, terms.

At the same time, the blinking light testifies to the repetition of a kind of fort/da game (Freud, 1920), by which he makes an attempt at managing fears of separation, to reassure himself of his capacity for loss and reunion. Being shipwrecked thus becomes a necessity; encountering the trauma with such extreme violence sets the conditions for questioning everything and revisiting the suffering aspects of the self, those that have not been sufficiently reassured by a qualitatively fulfilling relationship with the primary object (Winnicott, 1957). By its very nature, analysis proposes the trauma again, forcing the patient undertake the journey to recover the 'shipwrecked' part of the self, as happens with many patients who end up on the analyst's couch, suffocated by the glitter of a life filled to overflowing with possessions, but devoid of that sense of time and freedom of movement that enables affective contact. Such patients are isolated behind a barrier that is at first defensive, but that later becomes an insurmountable obstacle, as we see with the film's main character. This makes it impossible to 'let oneself go' in more demanding and rewarding affective relationships. The psychological obstacle to be surmounted, which wounds and draws blood, is represented vividly in the film by a jagged coral reef. The hero can only face this challenge by summoning up his remaining inventiveness and creativity. Far from being produced by magic or maniacal reparation of the object, the raft he makes requires hours and hours of work, a metaphor for the interminable hours of analytical labour that are required for working through.

The film portrays well the moments of mortal danger, the traumatic event (air crash) and, later, the risky crossing of the protective barrier (coral reef). Chuck may face the journey back towards life and relationships only if he accepts the risk of encountering again a love object that no longer needs to be maniacally repaired. Now, he may also cope with a benign regression (Balint, 1979[1959]), which, however, entails moments of mortal danger. Deeply moving because of its narcissistic suffering is the distancing and abandonment of the retreated area of the self, which is represented by the atoll, and the need to expose oneself to something that may be psychically fatal. Having crossed the coral reef, the raft drifts away from the atoll. Contemplating it from a distance, the castaway is then moved with a yearning nostalgia for that semblance of life that protected him from the awareness towards which he is now moving. It is an awareness of the likelihood of again being exposed to the trauma of loss and consciousness of time lost, spent in that suspension of affective life.

A similar feeling is often expressed in analysis; once the old defences have been abandoned, the affective distance enables the perspective to be adjusted, thus imposing the inexorable realisation of the illusionary nature of the neurotic devices. Another highly dangerous event in the quest for survival in *Castaway* is the loss of "the secret sharer," represented by the dummy Wilson. There is a high risk of malignant regression (Balint, 1979[1959]), a calling back to exposure to a primary/maternal object that looks on with indifference and does nothing. He is like a newborn baby lying next to an enormous object/mother (the whale that swims at the side of the raft), a mother who no longer carries him in her womb; she has expelled him, does not hold him in her arms or console him or feed him.

This is the abyssal silence, the silent scream (Bion, 1970), when the human voice is no more than the breathing of a primordial animal, an enigmatic place outside the sensory relation of the warm embrace, which the body surface is aware of long before it becomes "*moi peau*" (Anzieu, 1985). The sound comes from a baffling abyss, and the presence is that of an enormous being, made distant and incomprehensible, still almost inanimate because warmth and love are missing. In that scene, the risk of psychic death is extremely high; the castaway is at the crossroads of life and death, between negative and positive. The risk appears again when the body of the whale is replaced by the rusty hull of an enormous, silent cargo ship, which passes him by. For an instant, it appears to be deserted, piloted by a machine, the model of the primordial, affectless relation of the self, mechanical, hidden, and half-extinguished.

The individual who comes back to life after being cast away is now underweight, a corporal metaphor of internal suffering and transformation. He has to face the realisation that he has lost part of his life, both in terms of time and affection: he has lost his beloved Kelly. His fiancée, too, has left part of her life unresolved. She did not graduate but went along with what was suggested to get over the trauma and bereavement. Chuck gives her back her grandfather's watch, to which he has no further right, as it marked a bond with her that he must give up. He rightly, however, keeps her faded photograph, which belongs to him just like the tale of his desperation (his attempted suicide) and the memory of his solitude on the atoll, which he can now confide to a friend, who understands his grief and loss. He can express his gratitude to Kelly for keeping him company, then he can leave her and face an uncertain future.

In the film's unresolved conclusion, perhaps we glimpse a contemporary man's recognition and awareness that the great conquests and certainties of Robinson Crusoe are no longer his. Chuck Nolan knows that he must complete his task, be it large or small, by delivering the parcel that he did not open on the atoll, because, having a task, not grand, and also somewhat diminished, helped to save his life. At the end of the film, he finds himself at the crossroads, a place charged with oedipal significance. And here we leave him, with a close-up of the puzzled and enigmatic expression on Tom Hanks's face. Perhaps, this hints at the gaining of an authentic dimension of the self and relations. It is not a happy ending, contrary to classic Hollywood style. The director's camera and the inventiveness of the scriptwriter, for brief moments of fantasy, penetrate the very crevices where unconscious impressions lie concealed. Cinema reconfirms its interweaving with psychoanalysis and its role as a source to re-explore the echoes of half-extinguished or retreated parts of the self, because both psychoanalysis and cinema speak the unexpectedly intrusive language of the unconscious (Gabbard, 1997).

The effects of trauma: *The Secret of Their Eyes*[2] by Juan José Campanella

The plot

Based on the novel by Edoardo Sacheri, the action is set in 1974, just before the military coup in Argentina. The country is on the brink of dictatorship, one that will pervert justice and society in a reversal of values. Chaos and violence will prevail and some people, both victims and persecutors, will remain entrapped for ever. This is the political-historical background of this beautiful film, a thriller and a story of love and hate, revenge and regeneration, whose complexity intertwines different levels, from the public to the private.

The film tells the story of Benjamin Esposito (Ricardo Darin), a retired inspector of the Buenos Aires Court of Justice, who now, 25 years later, wants to write a novel on the unresolved rape and murder of a young bride, Liliana Coloto (Carla Quevedo).

At that time, thanks to the widower Ricardo Morales (Pablo Rago), to the judge, Irene Hastings (Soledad Villamil), Benjamin's secret love, and to his alcoholic colleague Pablo Sandoval (Guillermo Francella), he was able to arrest the murderer, Isidoro Gomez (Javier Godino). However, the military junta released Gomez in order to recruit him in the anti-subversive death squads. Despite this, and as a result of the perverse situation created by the dictatorship, the widower, who had waited an entire year for the killer to show up at the railway station, was able to capture him and claim that he had killed him. In fact he imprisoned him in an isolated country place, where he himself had moved and made him pay for his brutal crime, day after day, in the name of a justice he himself decreed. The cold case of Liliana Coloto still torments Benjamin, as does his secret love for Irene. Unable to resolve their differences in both social status and personality, they had separated, but now they meet again when life games are over: Irene is married to the man her family considered most suitable and Benjamin has spent a lifetime in a frontier town in a sort of suspended animation, mired in love affairs, with affects and memories too painful to be worked through, such as the violent death of his friend Pablo, killed in his place by the death squad and with an unresolved passion toward Irene.

The first image that appears, as the opening titles roll, will remain imprinted on the spectators' retina, and it will accompany them for the rest of the film, just as it remained in the mind of the protagonist: a pretty young woman, raped and murdered (a whole nation violated and torn?), a youth, like many other Argentinians in those years, without a future, lives taken away forever. The audience is captured by the images in the trauma-enhanced sensorial dimension, just as Benjamin is profoundly affected by something that begins to disrupt the absent-minded, light-hearted routine of his boring days.

Around the traumatic dimension narrated in the film, there is a male universe focusing on the main character: Pablo Sandoval, the alcoholic colleague; Ricardo Morales, the widower, and Isidoro Gomez, the murderer. The women protagonists are first, Liliana Coloto, the victim, whose memory awaits justice and reparation, and second, Irene Hastings, the judge. Each one of them is a fragmented, dissociated part of the spectator's and of Benjamin's Self, and it represents different understandings and interpersonal and intrapsychic knowledges of the affects moved in the story and of the grief the characters have been entrapped in.

Revenge and mourning

At the beginning of his novel *All That Is*, the American writer James Salter says, "There is a moment in life in which you realize that everything is a dream, and that only the things preserved by writing have a chance of being real" (Salter, 2013).

Benjamin Esposito could well subscribe to that statement, because through writing he attempts to find a way to revisit the traumatic events of his past life and to retrieve the voices of those who are absent (Freud, 1901), yet still so alive within.

The traumatic dimension is central in the film and in its characters, and it is repeated by means of an experience which is difficult to work through, highlighting the drama of loss and the intolerability of the affects linked to it. Benjamin's flashbacks are movingly nostalgic-like, for example, the sequence in which Irene follows the train that is taking Benjamin away. Another scene portrays a moment of daily routine, filled with love and tenderness, between Ricardo Morales and his wife. The two characters, Benjamin and Ricardo, obsessively repeat their traumatic experience, because by revisiting it in memory, despite the reactivation of painful loss, it will be, to a point, their only way to retrieve their history and not to lose their identity. It is their only hope, since they do not have a memory that can be shared, and they live in a solitude of affects, in a world without a future, full of nothing, as Morales often repeats, and as Benjamin himself is beginning to realize, as he is retiring, in a suspended affective dimension.

But from where should one begin? From the eyes of Irene, his lost love, as she runs after the train on which he is forced to leave in order to avoid being killed by the death squad, without having had the courage to ask her to go away with him? Or from the last breakfast of Liliana Coloto with her husband Ricardo Morales; a last, unforgettable breakfast, because it was full of the rich taste of life and love? Or, rather, from the rape, the trauma that has remained in their eyes? Benjamin and Ricardo are both paralyzed in a traumatic dimension.

Just as with analysis, the possibility of investigating past memories and unknown psychic territories requires a setting, in order to mobilize one's representational skills and allow remembering to unfold in a creative new reading in the present. The ability to experience mourning implies affective maturity, since the original mourning is at the basis of human psychism and of its health, making it possible to face potential future traumas.

However, denying or refusing to acknowledge its inevitability means that physical and psychic survival may be linked to the invention of a universe that swings from omnipotence to impotence, exposed to the repetition of a trauma, meant as a psychic event that does not modify. Once the transformative potentialities of memory and oblivion are blocked, the Ego re-experiences a state of *Hilflosigkeit*, that is, the inability to cope with an accumulation of internal and external excitements which are so powerful that, one might assume, they might bring about the laceration of the protective screen (Freud, 1925). On the contrary, the paradox that is implicit in the trauma itself, which "firstly, must not be forgotten, and secondly, must be forgotten" (Freud, 1934–38), can lead to a re-reading of the past, passing through the unresolved tangles of one's existence. Only thus can one then transform the negative, moving towards an area of shared enjoyment, where it is possible to rediscover the beauty of the object and of the Self, which was lost in the psychic rebellion against mourning (Freud, 1915). However, when the suffering overcomes one's own possibility of reparation, the awareness of having to cope with an impossible task paves the way to denial and to splitting in its most extreme forms, like revenge. The narcissistic wound that one has suffered is then reversed, by making the trauma enter the realm of omnipotence and of obsessional control (Goretti, 1997), reducing the object into a receptacle of its own psychic refuse, in a "perverse" dimension that shapes the other according to the needs of the subject. Morales, exposed to an unbearable loss, is "suspended" in the construction of a sophisticated revenge and will no longer be able to detach himself and really differentiate himself from the murderer, remaining imprisoned with him at Pata, an arid, place, a farm that is no longer productive.

For Benjamin, the possibility of working through mourning is in the writing of his novel, an idea that he pursues, despite Irene's ironical attack: "Why should you make your life more complicated? Why should you be so pathetic?"

On the contrary, Ricardo Morales, the widower, personifies the part of the trauma that cannot be worked through. He is "suspended" in the construction of a sophisticated form of revenge and will no longer be able to detach himself from the murderer: therefore he will remain engaged in a lifelong vendetta; a different kind of life sentence.

If revenge "is a kind of wild justice,"[3] Morales appears to obtain it through his actions, yet he is also despairing of it, considering the corruption of human justice in the country during that period. Morales replaces the traumatic abandonment he has suffered with the "indissolubility" of the sadomasochistic link which will bind him to his wife's rapist and murderer for the rest of his life. Thus, he will be able to control the killer omnipotently, as well as his lost object, transforming his longing for the lost object in an instrument for mutual control (Freud, 1919). To hate and punish Isidoro Gomez, is all he has. One could say that the shadow of the object falls on the enactment (Roussillon, 2015) of revenge: it lasts his entire life.

Memory, which begins from the here and now and then rewinds backwards, makes it possible to re-read events, according to the logic of affects, guiding Benjamin's memories on the basis of free associations, like in the course of an analysis, to reconstruct a story of destructive violence and passion, of guilt for the death of his friend Pablo, of distractions ("I was distracted for ten years"), and of denials, so as to avoid and eschew traumas and their recurring ghosts. For Ricardo Morales this is about an impossible working through mourning; memory is like a trauma that repeats itself, always the same, in an eternally identical representation of what has been lost.

Acknowledging the revengeful elements of his actions, might he have reached some sort of inner peace? And might this have allowed him to fulfil his desire for the multiplicity of life, thus overcoming the persecutory aspects of the search and the punishment of the killer, as well as the idealization of his lost wife? Actually, the wound suffered by his Self is an unbearable experience of loss concealing the destructiveness of a "nostalgia without object," as some authors put it (Andreoli, 1988), while others speak of "negative narcissism" (Green, 1983), of "black hole," of "nonsense" (Grotstein, 2007[1991]), of "blocked mourning" (Racamier, 1992).

We cannot forget, however, that those who should have dispensed justice have instead rewarded the criminal, subverting the laws of civil cohabitation and human piety. For Ricardo Morales, the daily, concrete renewal of an experience of contact with his wife's killer, despite its dramatic aspects, seems to be the only way he can retain his identity (Modell, 1984). Unable to share his memory with other human beings, he lives a clandestine, reclusive life, he indeed experiences complete solitude in terms of affects, in the dimension of a life suspended between sleep and waking, without dreams (Bion, 1962). The perspective of a future life is lost, time is flattened in a motionless "full of nothing" in the company of his mortal enemy, who concretely keeps him on the border of a psychic, unrepresentable, unspeakable void: the perceptive excitement, renewed in the daily care of his wife's killer is the only possibility for survival. Hate, existing before the object is invested, says Freud, hate that allows a surviving psychic functioning against psychic death, keeps him alive, even when the memory of his beloved wife starts to fade, as he tells Benjamin Esposito.

The film can be interpreted as the painful search for the protagonist's own identity: "I was distracted for twenty years, and now I have nothing to distract me," Benjamin says. He was distracted from looking into the wounded parts of his psyche, he was in denial, he lived in an excited dimension (a marriage, many affairs); but now this is no longer enough to distract his mind from that story, in which his fate was intertwined with the fate of so many other people.

Why now and not before? There is a limit to the amount of truth and reality that a human being can bear and sometimes only under special conditions, not to be overwhelmed, said T.S. Eliot (1943), and only now is Benjamin able to bear the truth of past events and bring them into awareness.

But still, why would a retired man, instead of quietly living out his final years, complicate his life by stirring up memories, traumas and passions once again? Why should he want to return to that troubling case?

Freud gives us the answer in "Mourning and Melancholia" (1915): working through mourning is something that complicates one's life, but to eschew it, to renounce the search for truth, switches off one's future, leading to a life without memories, without passion, full of nothing.

Still, experiencing passion can also complicate one's life, and I will discuss the importance of passion in a moment.

Benjamin returns to his old office in the austere and imposing court of Buenos Aires, because passions are difficult to experience and he needs to share them with someone, with Irene, who at first mocks him but then provides him with a writing tool, an instrument full of history and affects: an old Olivetti typewriter, with a faulty 'A' key, the right tool for rethinking their story.

From now on, Benjamin and Irene begin to function as a couple: one of the pair, alternatively, is always the carrier of passion, but that is the way a good couple may function; only one at a time in crisis (Kohut, 1971), while the other, in turn, keeps the passion alive. In life, as in analysis. When Benjamin appears to have given up, it is Irene who restarts the process, because they are aware that they have started talking to each other by means of the story of rape and murder that has affected them, because they loved each other, just as Morales loved his wife, and in his obsessional search for his wife's killer, he has kept his pure love alive, as Benjamin says.

There are many affects at play in the film: love, hate, revenge, possession, alternatively within knowledge and truth. Transformations take place in K, not in L or in H, as Bion reminds us (Bion, 1965). Passions arouse excitement, but without passion there is no true search. Passion is the affect of the true researcher, Benjamin, and his helpers, Pablo and Irene, while excitement is what stirs Isidoro, the murderer. Excitement fills one's emptiness for a moment, it keeps pain at a distance in order to avoid and deny it; Isidoro's eyes are always looking at Liliana in photos and his gaze reveals attraction, excitement, a wish for possession, obsessively linked to the object of his desire.

Pablo, Benjamin's alcoholic friend, understands it. He cannot cope with external reality and truth, he drowns in alcohol but with his altered and apparently bizarre imagination, he is capable of crossing the boundaries of common sense and going beyond. Irene, too, offers fundamental support in the unmasking of the murderer, allowing Benjamin to discover what goes on in the mind of a rapist and a killer. Irene, a woman, also a potential victim, it is she who understands the intrusive gaze of the rapist and knows how to challenge and break him down.

The character of Gomez represents the most primitive, revengeful and persecutory aspects of a personality, which must constantly be evacuated in the perverse and destructive possession of the object. Isidoro Gomez lives in a state of excitement in which he must act in order to evacuate beta elements (Bion, 1962). Indeed, he must keep increasing his dose of emotion, because if he attempted to stop, once the excitement is over, he would reveal his underlying catastrophic anxiety. His sense of fragmentation and imminent destruction turns into collusion and corruption of everything and everyone.

For this reason he can triumph in an upside-down world, perverted in its values, and become its ruthless instrument, completely enslaved by a power that overwhelms and destroys in order to survive, just as he is forced to do in order to fuel his negative narcissism, continuing to destroy and evacuate, thereby becoming a perfect war machine.

The analyst as a "true detective"

Someone wrote that Benjamin is a Marlowe-like, stubborn and solitary detective, who delves into the repressed aspects of Argentinian history between the death of Peron in 1974 and the deposition of Isabelita on behalf of General Videla, which marked the beginning of the fierce dictatorship in 1976.

I do not agree with this view. To me, Benjamin is, rather, the "True Detective" of the television series, crazed with love and solitude, able to act like a visionary when necessary, to abandon the reality principle to come to the solution; like the analyst who, confronted with the traumatic areas and in the face of denials of his analysand, tries to imagine and tolerate the unthinkable. Instead of memories he finds only "amnestic traces," that perhaps once affectively revitalized will again "search for representations" (Racalbuto, 1994) and perhaps they will find them. Benjamin, "the true detective," needs a partner able to cope with the weight of the truth, because there is no real investigation without passion, but the latter must be supported by a couple (any reference to the analytic couple is purely accidental!). But he is the one, however, who holds the story together, not only because he discovers the killer and solves the case, but also because he knows and understands Morales's pathological thoughts about revenge, and also because that is the only way for him to find his own internal resolution. Benjamin knows that the story is not over because he understands Morales and the depth of his wounds. He does not believe that Morales has truly given up the only wish he had to cope with his future: to find his wife's rapist and murderer and send him to prison for life.

Benjamin has the characteristics of the good detective (and of the good enough analyst), he is able to look too where it is forbidden to do so: breaking into the house of Gomez's aunt, searching for pictures and letters, confusedly looking at Irene's unexpectedly open blouse that fleetingly exposes her breasts, and noticing the killer's obsessive, fixed gaze upon them.

He is passionate, while Isidoro, the murderer, is excitable: while passion disrupts the balance of the Self, complicating, confounding and thus creating new links, excitement blocks thinking, evades it and moves towards action. However, passion and excitement are intertwined and indeed fuel one another. Excitement, as a state of the Self, is the sign of a deep wound, of an emptiness that the exciting object can fill only for a moment, while passion, instead, is a comprehensive state of the personality, "the soul's own motion," in the romantic imagination, and so it is something from which any possible change in the subject and in the world can proceed. Not a state of a soul's exaltation stirred by strong emotions, but rather the tense orientation of a consciousness that is aware of itself, bringing forth a project for change (Bion, 1965).

Unlike excitement, passion is intense but long lasting and rooted in the body; it tends towards action and may abuse reality (like the crazy idea of beginning the investigation from the killer's point of view) because it transforms reality into a sort of forge, using its materials and its details in order to reach its aim, namely truth.

Passion can keep one's object alive for twenty-five years, as it has for Benjamin and Morales, the widower. The latter, however, is moved by his own unworked-through mourning, something that his mind could not tolerate, not by love for truth. Hatred is the only passion left in him. Can there really be a passionate search without a resolution? The film does not answer this question and it has an open ending: the passion of Irene and Benjamin will be "complicated," but they will not renounce it or their quest for truth; the resolution of some traumatic losses seems to be impossible.

Benjamin leaves Morales and Gomez in the prison at Pata and he goes towards a new life, complicated as that may be. He leaves and accepts the limits of his investigation and research, he understands that there are no possible solutions because Gomez and Morales are in some way both carriers of an "absolute sorrow/grief", of a trauma that has torn their subjectivities.

The end of the film compels us to face the limit of the analysability of the real trauma.

"History", writes the Italian psychoanalyst, Lucio Russo (2008, p. 12), "teaches that in the course of the individual and collective history 'absolute traumas' happen (Shoah, genocides, massacres). These absolute traumas run the risk not to be incorporated and metabolized by psychic systems, they are instead evacuated, denied and as cursed remains they come back in delusional states, nightmares, panic and anxiety attacks." To these, I add the destructiveness that comes again and again in the course of history.

Benjamin, the key character of the film, in the prison of Pata, sees the "horror" of the absolute trauma, he does not judge, but he has no concrete solution to offer, therefore he turns over a new leaf. He leaves the spectators with the idea that the passionate loving research for truth helped him to integrate his affects from *odi et amo* to *temo/te amo*.

Our hope as researchers in psychoanalysis is that traumas, individual and collective, find the way towards symbolization, becoming memories that can be shared, that they are made human by someone who does not petrify in front of them, as we analysts try to achieve in our clinical practice.

After the war: *The Third Man* by Carol Reed

The film library of Bologna, as it continues to enhance the history of cinema with the restoration of masterpieces, is winning more and more well-deserved fame at an international level. Recently, it restored *The Third Man*, a film by Carol Reed with unforgettable performances by Orson Welles, Joseph Cotten and Alida Valli – or "Valli" as she is listed in the opening credits – and Trevor Howard, who is supported by other character actresses of the highest level. The restored version renders the contrasts of the vintage black and white to the fullest, letting us enjoy Robert Krasker's photography to the utmost, as it is accompanied by Anton Karas's ultra-famous music and the voices of the original version.

The story is familiar, but is subject to repression … So, a brief review to refresh one's memory may be useful. In 1946, Holly Martins arrives in Vienna, still in ruins following the end of the war, and still divided into occupation zones. He is an American writer of westerns, sent there by his childhood friend, Harry Lime, who – however – has just been killed in a suspicious accident. In fact, some witnesses describe two men who were at the scene of the accident, others mention three. This is where "the third man" comes from. Lime is, in fact, alive and wanted by the allied police, the Americans, for smuggling adulterated penicillin which has caused, and continues to cause, a terrible death among many children. In this way, Martins discovers an unexpected truth about his childhood friend; he gets to know Lime's girlfriend, too. She is indebted to Lime for her clandestine expatriation from Czechoslovakia, which had already been invaded by the Russians at that time. And for this she continues to be grateful, even in the face of evidence regarding unsavoury trafficking for profit, and of his having become a perverse, destructive person.

In a gloomy, baroque, anguished, expressionist Vienna, Orson Welles inhabits one of the most contemptible characters in film, making him – still today – a kind of keenly fascinating non-hero. A panoply of factors – atmosphere and cut of the framing, close-ups of suspicious faces, a camera which rummages through cars and around doors, beneath street lamps and the unforgettable theme played repetitively on the zither by Anton Karas – seduces us into following the story and seems to suggest an eternity of a carousel of human existence and of the world; it is a panoply of factors which makes the movie an undisputed masterpiece.

I have seen the film at various times of life, yet still, the pleasure is priceless, starting with the trailer which introduces the film, all the way to the end credits which accompany us as we leave the theatre, along with the enthusiastic comments of cinemagoers of various ages, and the dream-like atmosphere we have been immersed in for the duration of the film.

Many people experience a sensation that they have seen the film before, even if they only realize at a certain point in the showing that they actually have seen it already. Usually, memory is reactivated in the minor scenes: a friend tells me she remembered the plot only when she saw the scene in which Anna (Valli)'s kitten curls up at Lime's (Welles's) feet, when although believed dead he reappears for the first time, in the recessed entrance of a building. Others remember the parrot biting the escaping Holly (Cotten), and how every time he says he was pecked by a parrot he will be taken for crazy or drunk, heightening the scene's comic effect. Still others remember the unpleasant, lying child (innocence contaminated and perverted by war) who accuses Holly of being the murderer of the doorman, an inconvenient witness. Everyone, or almost everyone, seems to remember the unforgettable quip of the cynical Lime who tries to justify his choice to stay on the side of evil in order to get rich, to perversely break the law, manipulating external and internal realities, bending them toward his corrupt ends.

All of us, those who belong to the generation immediately following the war years, find again here the adults of our childhood; we all recognize the leanness, the gestures, the clothes, the hairstyles. From the depths of our memories of what we really saw in childhood mixed with what we became familiar with through photo archives and documentary films, we see again the devastated, semi-deserted cities our parents, grandparents, aunts and uncles moved though. We breathe with verisimilitude the climate of those who had just emerged from war, totalitarian regimes, the Shoah.

Looking at the film, we are set down in an atmosphere which has all the shades of repressed memories, of the Oedipal story we each carry inside, the "third one" we always struggle to identify or allow entry to our awareness: this is where the cover-up memories come in (the particulars of the cinematographic story which stick in our minds and the continuous repression effect which seems to connect this historical masterpiece to the imagination, in all of us). So Holly becomes each one of us: he is innocent, naive – like the children who look out curiously at the adult world, at desire – represented by the stunning Anna, as enigmatic as the Sphinx. The infused myths of childhood and adolescence regarding parental figures, regarding the ones we have loved, give way in the face of an eruption of impulses.

There is more, however. There is the trauma from which everything and everyone – people, things, landscapes, animate and inanimate objects – has just emerged, with their sentiments and their subjectivity. Everything appears to us as the dawn of a world on the rebound, ready to be reborn, beginning with the distinction between what is dead and what is not (Is Lime dead or not?), of what is good and what is evil in this character – the third man. It is an extraordinary invention, an unforgettable representative of evil, of the dark side which lodges in each human being, which can always resurface. It may be capable of any atrocity: of the unthinkable murder of children, the apex of innocence, the vital part of the psyche; and it can contaminate, even infect the medicine, the drug (penicillin) which cures and restores life. In this sense, the screenwriter and director succeed at giving a representation of that unfathomable, negative element of the human psyche, always at war against life, an element so deeply complicated by the horrors of the Second World War. The final scene of the film is set in the cemetery where Lime has just been buried. However, we cannot celebrate fully in the rebirth of life, nor do we know what path the two protagonists must take, if they will live "happily ever after" – as every self-respecting fairy tale should end – giving life to a couple which lays anew foundations for the world, or if their paths will continue in opposite directions.

As occurs around the chasm which a collective trauma like war creates, fragments of memory remain – minute screens, which are impressed on our mind – while the totality of the story slips away, along with its profound meaning.

In the climate of a traumatized Europe, just emerging from the horror of war, from the trauma, an improbable character falls into the story: a certain Joseph Cotten. He is young – just like the other main and supporting characters in the film – naive, childish with an innocent affectivity, rudimentary in his pursuit of a truth and justice which the adult world seems to have forgotten with its deceitful manipulations of truth and various perversions. He is an American cowboy, a writer of westerns – certainly no devotee of James Joyce and the "stream of consciousness," of which he knows absolutely nothing, as seems clear in the exhilarating sequence of the culture club conference. It is one of the film's lighter scenes, which is a priceless medley of lightness and drama, thriller and melodrama. A true masterpiece of cinema rediscovered.

Note

1 A previous version of this chapter was published in the *International Journal of Psychoanalysis* (2003), 84(1): 169–172.
2 Published in the *International Journal of Psychoanalysis* (2007) 95(5): 1483–1491.
3 Francis Bacon, "Of Revenge" (1597), quoted in R. Speziale-Bagliacca (1997), *Colpa:* Considerazioni su Rimorso, Vendetta e Responsabilità.

References

Andreoli, Antonio. 1988. "Le Moi et son Objet narcissique." In *Acts del 48° Congrès des Psychanalystes de langue française des pays romans.* Champagne-sur-Sein: Imprimerie Cuesnon.

Anzieu, Didier. 1985. *Le Moi Peau.* Paris: Bordas.

Balint, Michael. 1979[1959]. *The Basic Fault.* London and New York: Routledge. Reprint by Enid Balint.

Bion, Wilfred R. 1962. *Learning from Experience.* London: William Heinemann.

Bion, Wilfred R. 1965. *Transformations: Changes from Learning to Growth.* London: William Heinemann.

Bion, Wilfred H. 1970. *Attention and Interpretation: A Scientific Approach to Insight in Psycho-Analysis and Groups.* London: Tavistock Publications.

Campanella, Juan José. (dir.) *El secreto de sus ojos.* [*The Secret in Their Eyes*] 2009. Argentina; Spain: Gran Via Productions, IM Global, Route One Films. Film.

Conrad, Joseph. 1982. *Heart of Darkness* [1902] and *The Secret Sharer* [1912]. London: Bantam.

Defoe, Daniel. 1996. *Robinson Crusoe.* New York: Barnes & Noble Books.

Eliot, T.S. 1943. "Burnt Norton." In *Four Quartets.* London: Faber & Faber.

Ferro, Antonino. 2010. *Tormenti di Anime. Passioni, Sintomi, Sogni* [*Soul Torments: Passions, Symptoms and Dreams*]. Milan: Raffaello Cortina.

Freud, Sigmund. 1901. "Fragment of an Analysis of Hysteria. Dora's Clinical Case." *Standard Edition, Vol. 7.* London: Hogarth Press, p. 3.

Freud, Sigmund. 1915. "Mourning and Melancholia." *Standard Edition, Vol. 14.* London: Hogarth Press, p. 239.

Freud, Sigmund. 1919. "A Child is being Beaten." *Standard Edition, Vol. 17.* London: Hogarth Press, p. 177.

Freud, Sigmund. 1920. "Beyond the Pleasure Principle." *Standard Edition, Vol. 18.* London: Hogarth Press, p. 7.

Freud, Sigmund. 1925. "Inhibition, Symptoms and Angst." *Standard Edition, Vol. 20.* London: Hogarth Press, p. 77.

Freud, Sigmund. 1934–38. "Moses and Monotheism." *Standard Edition, Vol. 23*. London: Hogarth Press, p. 3.

Gabbard, Glen. 1997. "The Psychoanalyst at the Movies." *International Journal of Psychoanalysis* 78(3): 429–434.

Goretti, Giovanna. 1997. "Le Menti Violate." *Rivista di Psicoanalisi* XLIII(4): 636–656. Rome: Borla.

Green, André. 1983. *Narcissisme de Vie, Narcissisme de Mort*. Paris: Les Edition des Minuit.

Grotstein, James S. 2007. *A Beam of Intense Darkness*. London: Karnac.

Kohut, Heinz. 1971. *The Analysis of the Self*. London: Hogarth Press.

Modell, Arnold H. 1984. *Psychoanalysis in a New Context*. London: The New Library of Psychoanalysis.

Ogden, Thomas H. 2004. "This Art of Psychoanalysis." *International Journal of Psychoanalysis* 85(4): 857–877.

Racalbuto, Agostino. 1994. *Tra il fare e il dire*. Milan: Raffaello Cortina Editore.

Racamier, Paul-Claude. 1992. *Le Génie des Origines*. Paris: Payot.

Reed, Carol. (dir.) *The Third Man*. 1949. London: British Lion Film Corporation. Film.

Riefolo, Giuseppe. 2015. *Il film di cinquanta minuti*. Turin: Antigone Edizioni.

Riolo, Fernando. 2018. "Il metodo psicoanalitico e i suoi funtori." In T. Bastianini and A. Ferruta (eds), *La cura psicoanalitica contemporanea*. Rome: Giovanni Fioriti Editore.

Roussillon, René. 2017. "Fondamenti e Processi dell'Incontro Psicoanalitico." In N. Rossi and I. Ruggiero (eds), *La Relazione Analitica*. Milan: Franco Angeli, pp. 44–50.

Russo, Lucio. 2008. "Evento e Psiche." In *Atti del Convegno. L'Impronta del Trauma. Sui Limiti della Simbolizzazione*. Rome: Astrolabio.

Salter, James. 2013. *All That Is*. New York: Penguin Random House, p. 12.

Speziale Bagliacca, Roberto. 1997. *Colpa. Considerazioni su Rimorso, Vendetta e Responsabilità*. Rome: Astrolabio.

Steiner, John. 1993. *Psychic Retreats*. London: Routledge.

Winnicott, Donald W. 1957. *The Child and the Family*. London: Tavistock Publications.

Winnicott, Donald W. 1992. *Collected Papers. Through Paediatrics to Psychoanalysis*. London: Institute of Psychoanalysis and Karnac.

Zemeckis, Robert. (dir.) *Castaway*. 2000. Los Angeles: 20th Century Fox. Film.

Chapter 4

In search of the lost father

My Architect. Different architectures of creativity: Louis and Nathaniel Kahn[1]

My Architect, nominated for an Oscar as the best documentary of 2004, is inscribed in the history of being one of those cinematographic gems that allow us to approach a great artist – in this case, the architect Louis Kahn – and to help us understand his work.

The film is also part of the history of the works produced by sons and daughters who, through the means of artistic expression, search for answers to the mysteries left behind by parents who were dramatically lost.[2] Their artistic works demonstrate the laborious process of working-through that accompanies reconstruction of memories that can offer meaning and provide consolation for traumatic loss.[3]

The death of a parent is one of the most painful and incomprehensible events for a child's psyche while it is still in formation and it forces him to undergo the complex working through of a number and variety of affects that include, often in conflict with one another, the following: sorrow, anger, guilt, hate as a reaction to sudden abandonment, and ambivalence between the desire to live and the desire to reunite with the loved object, as emphasized by authors starting with Freud (1915), to our present time (Ogden, 2004).

Rather than opening the way to creativity, mourning can represent a formidable obstacle to the development of the capacity to fantasize, removing libidinal energy and vigour from spontaneity and curiosity, and inhibiting the expression of emotionality. Many studies confirm, however, that pain can influence and can almost demand the establishment of processes that make play and fantasy possible – processes that can be, in that sense, the basis of creativity, posing the question of the relationship between the pain of loss and artistic expression.

Creativity, understood as an affirmation of the full, individual capacity to fantasize and to give life to forms of representation that can be shared and communicated, seems therefore to act as a powerful antidote, like an element that propels one towards renewal, in order to again set in motion the symbolic and representative processes that were interrupted or inhibited by an absence of the working through of mourning.

So says David Aberbach (1989) in examining literary works about survivors of the Holocaust and comparing them with those by persons exposed to individual mourning. The aim of his work is to demonstrate the role of creativity as an individual and collective response to mourning, in considering that, while clinical studies show us the universality of reactions to loss brought about by death, creative responses remind us of the singularity of every state of mourning. He adds in his conclusion that creativity may be a means through which the individual in mourning, whether grief stems from a normal cause or from collective trauma, can express his pain and master it, thereby restoring meaning to his life.

Continuing on the topic of the connecting points between loss and death, mourning and creativity, Maria Luisa Algini (2009) perceives an internal push to be creative, which she revealingly calls "the obstinate path of creativity," activated to counteract the risk of psychic death, of being immobilized and affectively frozen.

The artist and the person occupied in the working through of mourning behave in a way that is not dissimilar on a psychic level, in order to restabilize the emotional earthquake provoked by the physical loss, urged onward by the necessity of finding a way out, of opening a passage for oneself – although a painful and perhaps only a partial one – towards the future. Through representation after representation, these persons mount a slow, exploratory march toward the edge of the incomprehensible "abyss" created by the loss, without being engulfed by it, and in fact find consolation in the construction of an object re-created from fantasy.

Sons and daughters who work through artistic means to interpret and understand the mystery left within by a parent who was dramatically lost, like Nathaniel Kahn, are probably spurred on by the necessity of going forward in order to gain a future that is not blocked by the traumatic event, together with the need to prevent the total loss of the loved object, re-creating through sublimation and art the parent whom they did not know and who was lost too soon and so inexplicably.

The vestige of the loved parent that they have kept within themselves, which has survived the storms of rage, of destruction, and the demand to be liberated from the dead/killed object that inhabited them, becomes the spark for the creation of a "dreamed" relationship with the object, in which there can be a renewed illusion of coming closer to the blessed state that the loved presence bestowed, without giving up in the face of disappointment.

In the flow of images in Nathaniel Kahn's short film, we witness a determined and "obstinate" search for information on the father and his work. In sequence after sequence, interview after interview, the impossible solution to the inherent paradox of the working through of mourning – that is, keeping the tie to the lost object without being blocked by it – becomes the impetus for the search and the creative drive.

In the case of Nathaniel Kahn, the choice of a visual, cinematographic medium reaches its *raison d'être* in the graphic and figurative skills utilized by Louis Kahn in his work and in playing with his son, but perhaps also in the extraordinary force of the visual impact that his architectural monuments communicate, as I will try to show in what follows.

The search for data and its collection: information about Louis Kahn's life

The title *My Architect*, chosen for this short, poetic film by the director Nathaniel Kahn, emphasizes the interweaving of different levels of the public and private (Capuano, 2006). The first level concerns Louis Kahn, one of the foremost architects of the twentieth century, and the second, a son who is trying to understand the father who died suddenly when he was eleven years old. The process of remembering, in which the director purposely involves the viewer, starts from the diligent collection of pieces of information about the famous man who was his father, through interviews and documents.

The chosen sequence of images, even though utilized in a documentary film, does not follow a chronological order but rather an associative principle, one whose underlying rationale must be sought in the "affective truth" that Nathaniel – already an established director – casts in the form of a cinematographic account. We are made to participate in this account in a close interweaving between historical/documentary truth and reconstruction/narrative fiction (Golinelli, 2004).

The film begins with the short newspaper article that announced the death of Louis Kahn in New York's Penn Station on 17 March 1974. The body was transported to a morgue and identified only three days later, since it appeared that all personal information had been removed from the documents on his person. Nathaniel and his mother – who were not mentioned in the public obituary since the relationship was extramarital – learned only later of the death of their loved one, and could not attend the funeral or see the lifeless body for a final goodbye.

One must keep in mind the attitudes of respectability and convention in the American middle class during the post-World War II era, glimpsed in some of the interviews of the time, in order to understand – apart from Louis Kahn's personal characteristics – the atmosphere of secrecy in his complicated romantic life.

Louis Kahn was married to Esther Israeli, a neurologist who had been for some time the family's real economic support, and the father of a daughter, Sue Ann. Louis also had amorous relationships with two of his collaborators and colleagues: Anne Tyng, the mother of his daughter Alexandra, and Harriet Pattison, Nathaniel's mother. He never divorced his wife, who seems not to have suspected anything of her husband's extramarital relationships; his three children did not know of each other's existence until the director Nathaniel Kahn began his investigation.

There is a tightly bound affective logic in Nathaniel's decision to begin his reconstruction at the very end, from the place where his father died. The death of a loved one is a heartrending event, linked to the disappearance of the other with all that characterizes his bodily, physical presence. For Nathaniel, the working through of mourning must start out from a "physically" recovered place: the anonymous underground train station and the unknown person who found the body, whom the director tracks down with some difficulty twenty-five years later, and whom he interviews.

That unidentified body, lost in the crowded Penn Station, calls to mind the sad fate of an outcast, a poor man without documents in a society that considers poverty an unequivocal sign of existential failure. In retrospect, the finale of his existence gives a dramatic flavour to the life of Louis Kahn; it has almost the meaning of an inevitable, forced return to the trauma of his arrival in the United States, as experienced by the four-year-old son of Estonian immigrants at the beginning of the 1900s.

To venture a more unformulated hypothesis, that death could be the suicidal choice of a man who, while struggling with his most imposing work – the Bangladesh Parliament, certainly the work that occupied him for the longest time up until the end of his life[4] – was also plagued by debts, despite fame and international success, and now found himself anticipating the catastrophe of a major affective change that was impossible for him: that is, the act of leaving his first and only wife, the woman who had represented a secure anchor for him over time, in order to choose a new family, Nathaniel and his mother. He had promised them this and they expected that he would follow through. The deleted documents could in fact bear out a hypothesis of a desire to disappear and never be found again.

The interviews

In the film, we see images in sequence from Louis Kahn's repertoire: he strolls around the university campus; he poses with Nathaniel during one of the weekly visits made to the boy and his mother in the evenings, before returning home to his wife; pictures of the young Louis as a student, together with his school companions; and of Louis as a child with his parents or in the arms of his mother. These images alternate with interviews with celebrated architects – Philip Johnson, Vincent Scully, I.M. Pei, Frank Gehry[5] – all among the most eminent figures in twentieth-century architecture. These colleagues and friends, having known Kahn directly, speak to his uncommon qualities of freedom and intellectual honesty as an architect among the very best. Some of them loved and admired their brilliant colleague, while others had been in conflict with him or had envied him, perhaps feeling themselves as the "losing parties" before his genius – to use Thomas Bernhard's (1983) expression.

In the flow of cinematographic images, we revisit, together with Nathaniel, the portrait of a man considered to be one of the great masters of architecture in the twentieth century,[6] during the Golden Age of an epoch dominated by ingenious innovators such as Le Corbusier, Mies van der Rohe, and Walter Gropius. But this era also encompassed the Great Depression, a time of struggle against unemployment and economic problems; and as the son of very poor immigrants, Kahn was marked by a deprived childhood.

Perhaps this autobiographical information partially justifies the judgement of his contemporaries: that Kahn was a man of great talent, rich in idealism and spirituality, a fine teacher, but that his methods were often anachronistic, inappropriate, and anti-conformist, and he had very little business sense. He was fundamentally isolated, even after his gifts were generally recognized. Only at the age of fifty did he begin to be recognized, after an award from the American Academy in Rome (1950–51), which indicated a definite turning point in his way of thinking about architecture.

In the next twenty-five years and up until his death, Louis Kahn did not stop questioning himself about the essence of architecture, and he constructed and planned many buildings, having in mind and before his eyes the many ancient civilizations he had seen and reproduced in his beautiful sketches of Egyptian, Greek, and Roman ruins. Admiration for the monumentality and timelessness of architectural motifs like pyramids, dolmens, and columns, and love for materials like time-resistant bricks, used alongside modern materials, became leading characteristics of his work, transforming it forever. That probably distanced him from his contemporaries, both functionalists and modernists,[7] who spoke of lightness, transparency, and movement, while Kahn rediscovered monumentality, durability, and the robust nature and strength of the architecture of the past.

In this short film, shots of his most celebrated and discussed works pass by in turn and alternate with each other: the many works that were not accomplished and those that he brought to completion, mixed with verbal accounts from people whom he met on a more personal level than as an architect –taxi drivers, for example, who drove him in his frenetic movements between building sites, as well as between his three "families." As a child, Nathaniel, too, rode in those taxis together with his mother when, after a happy evening, they separated from Kahn, who returned to his legitimate family in the heart of the night.

The director then films his meetings with the women who loved his father, two of whom challenged the conventions of the time, the conformity of North American society and of Jewish culture of that era. The film shows his father's face disfigured by burns sustained in childhood – and, even more "burning," his betrayals and abandonings. The approach toward this painful truth about his father is a testimony to deeply rooted and tenacious work on Nathaniel's part, the work of gathering together the few available details on his celebrated parent in order to create new connections, to fill the holes in his data and in his memory, thus rewriting the private history of an illicit, secret son.

The cinematographic and the internal setting

As mentioned earlier, the pain and loss that accompany the death of a dearly loved person are part of universal experience, but the intensity and quality of that experience are in some measure completely private and unique for each of us, "creative" in that sense.

Nathaniel unveils for the viewer only a part of his task of working through, the part that he completed with the expressive capacities of an adult who manages his medium with competence, the movie camera that has furnished him with eyes able to penetrate and revisit the mystery that lacerated his childhood, giving him the right degree of distance from which to travel backwards through his family history.

In revisiting with a movie camera the buildings designed and constructed by his father, he creates a cinematographic setting, which permits him to find an "internal" setting appropriate for directing his goal – "like a light beam" – toward that mental place where the characters and scenes of his deepest and most meaningful life move about. The screen becomes the vehicle that places the object in an intermediate space, not too concrete yet not too illusory, and is precisely this that allows one to gain access to otherwise unapproachable emotions.

Recovery of the deepest dimension of this space and of the buildings themselves assumes the meaning, in Nathaniel's movie, of reviving the imaginary place in which pleasure and pain, union and separation, can be re-experienced in an affective continuity that permits him to tolerate and experience the bliss of rediscovery and the anguish of separation.

His father's rediscovered architecture – thanks also to its concrete quality, perhaps, and the visual impact it can provoke – becomes a place of fusion and of loss, where Nathaniel can repair the wounds inflicted by the anger caused by the legitimate, desperate need to defend himself against senseless loss. Thus the architectural space becomes the psychic space in which new affective and creative dimensions are opened up. The visual space, revived by Nathaniel's goal, is enriched by the emotional story of the characters involved, and this in turn evokes emotional fascination in the viewer.

Intrigued, we follow the movie camera that Nathaniel places between himself and the object to create a distance that permits him to come closer, and we linger with him over the faces of his father's students, genuinely impressed and admiring of Louis's anti-conformist teaching and his passion for architecture. Through their eyes the son seems to see his father's ingenuity from an adult vantage point, to see him as an innovator capable of transmitting enduring knowledge, in his own way the creator of a continuity between past, present, and future – a continuity that was re-created and extended by his architectural works. Nathaniel's gaze is thus enriched by the same spellbound admiration that the students demonstrate, recognizing this as an appropriate feeling when confronted with such genius.

Each one of the people who appear in the short film is engaged in his own "journey" of working through the loss: some mourn the great architect; some see him as a valuable friend, they admire him for his capacity to dream, and others see him as an over-endowed rival. And it is precisely the concerted nature of this tribute to Louis's memory that the director observes and recaptures, because that allows him to be reflected in the grief and other affects of others, now that Nathaniel can reveal his identity and thus, share their pain, which he might not have been able to do earlier.

This new form of shared consolation supports him in going on to "complicate" his life in order to remember and understand twenty-five years after his father's disappearance, that he can now no longer content himself with the truth that up until that moment was enough for him.

And it does complicate his life – showing us his retrospective journey through memory, making us live it together with him through images, words spoken and written by his father, the persons, the objects, the buildings that function as "thing presentations" reactivating the "word presentations." These traces of his father, charged with affectivity, are imbued with his physical presence, revisited in the flesh (Racalbuto, 1994). From these Nathaniel begins to reconstruct a knowledge previously impeded by pain, and he pushes himself to the point of that internal and external silence in which – according to the architect Doshi, with whom Louis Kahn spent the day before his death – he will rediscover his father and will understand his mysteries, his greatness, and his profound humanity.

Louis's architecture and that of Nathaniel

If, for the father, "architecture doesn't exist. Only the work of an architect exists" (Braghieri, 2005, p. 87), then the son is offering us his "architecture" of his father, reconstructed in the beautiful imagery that the paternal works are based on. The eyes of the child/adult son look at these works, enchanted, moving in spaces between buildings that appear to us like a photographic transcription of a play space, given to him by his father – despite the absences, the broken promises, the escapes into an adult reality that was often incomprehensible to the eyes of a child.

The poetry of images and that of architecture blend creatively, and the material from which Nathaniel's story originates gives form to a new sequence, affectively enriched, in which Louis Kahn's buildings gain even more thickness and depth, if that is possible, and reveal their spirituality, which is one of the most noble characteristics of his work.

Architectural spaces must possess an evocative capacity, and for Nathaniel, who sets about listening to the profound message in his father's constructions, they acquire it. When we see him skating on the pavement of the Salk Institute in San Diego, which opens out on the Pacific Ocean, we experience with him the recovered symbolic dimension of the meaning of his father's absence. His father makes himself present and alive through the spaciousness, the geometrical forms, the light, shadow, water, and sky.

He skates in a timeless dimension, reinventing a childhood game in the space marked out by a building that could be an enormous Lego construction, assembled together with his father, the builder of castles, of enchanted palaces, where Louis located the fairy tales that he recounted to Nathaniel. He thus resumes skating in a "paternal" space, circumscribed by the buildings, where he achieves a transformation brought about by his personal working through: the space crisscrossed by enlivened affects takes on a symbolic dimension, permitting the repetition of "The exciting and silent experience of childhood, of being the other and of passing the other, of being distinct, separate, but of placing oneself in relation" (Augé, 2005).

The artistic architectural object embodies, then – for us viewers, too – a father who is different from the historical one who was encountered and lost, and introduces the one who, at the end of the journey, Nathaniel will discover inside himself. "Thanks to this trip, my father became real," he will say at the end of the film, no longer referring to the dreamed father, the idealized one, "hated" for his human weakness, but the father who left an ingenious legacy, a monumental one. One could say, quoting another comment of Louis Kahn: "Monumentality in architecture can be understood as a spiritual quality that makes the eternal character of the construction explicit" (quoted by Braghieri, p. 19).

"A good building, a marvellous ruin"

"A good building would produce a marvellous ruin" is a famous remark of Louis Kahn's, dense and complex, like his legacy as architect and man. I like to think that Nathaniel may have reflected at length on this comment, in which one can catch the self-assurance of a builder-innovator who rediscovers a new confidence in solid materials, experienced "in the flesh" through the contemplation and study of the ruins of antiquity, and who understands their strength.

In a letter written to his co-workers from Rome on 6 December 1950, Kahn wrote:

> I am definitely realizing that the architecture of Italy will remain the source of inspiration for future works. Whoever doesn't see it this way should look at it again. Our things seem little by comparison: here all the pure forms are experienced in all the variations of architecture.
>
> (Braghieri, p. 20)

In a metaphorical vein, we can hear the self-confidence of one who has used "good" materials in his romantic relationships as well, and in the love for his heirs, his son and daughters.

In this comment, there is a sense of the transience of human things and of the very human effort aimed at overcoming the inexorable passage of time, at conquering oblivion and decadence. Vestiges of the self-regard of a genius are also there – the products of an awareness of leaving behind something strong, great, constructed with passion, both in his works and in his heirs; the first of these are understood and loved by his students and by those who constructed buildings after him, and the second are capable of embracing an inheritance of mixed emotionality.

There is also a love for beauty in that remark, for that mysterious, enigmatic reaction rooted deeply in all of us, the beauty of buildings designed and built by an architect who knew how to exist somewhat outside the conventions of his time, in order to pursue his own innovative and brilliant ideas. All this is rediscovered and exalted by the images that Nathaniel puts into place in his film. However, in Louis Kahn's comment there is also a denial of the ineluctable destruction of materials, a complex theme to which I will return.

Transience

The perception of beauty is inevitably accompanied by nostalgia and an awareness of the transience to which human things are destined, as Freud writes in the opening lines of his beautiful essay of 1915.

> Not long ago I went on a summer walk through a smiling countryside in the company of a taciturn friend and of a young but already famous poet. The poet admired the beauty of the scene around us but felt no joy in it. He was disturbed by the thought that all this beauty was fated to extinction, that it would vanish when winter came, like all human beauty and all the beauty and splendour that men have created or may create. All that he would otherwise have loved and admired seemed to him to be shorn of its worth by the transience which was its doom.
>
> (Freud 1915, p. 305)

In that essay, Freud makes reference to the "revolt in … [our] minds against mourning" (ibid., p. 306), as an experience that depreciates the enjoyment of the beautiful and impedes our regaining possession of it. This can occur to the point that the recovered capacity to tolerate the permeation of contradictory emotions and affects that bind us to the loved object will not permit a return to living, that is, to hopefulness and to suffering, and to enjoying a reconstructed wholeness.

The disavowal of what has been lost can follow many paths: it can make one insensitive to love and beauty, or it can nourish a compulsive idealization, object by object and love by love, as was the case for Kahn's father, one might say. In fact, his creativity seems to be tied to the continual re-creation and reparation of a self in search of the image of what was traumatically lost: perhaps an unresolved, transgenerational remainder of being exiled, or of the intact skin of a child permanently burned by hot embers, which he had wanted so much to get close to that he had been burned. In that event he was sustained by the powerful love of his mother – who, after the accident, said that he would become a great man, while his father said that he would have preferred him to die! (Braghieri, 2005).

Among the earliest memories that Nathaniel confesses to having felt resurfacing, at a certain point in his cinematographic account, is the sound of his father's voice and the contact with his burned skin: the child actually loved to make his father repeat the story of that traumatic event. There are traumas – especially collective ones, as has been noted – that require more than a generation to be faced up to and tolerated; and emigration, which the Kahn family was forced to undertake, is certainly one of these. The remains of unresolved mourning, the splits, make Louis's repetitive push to "create" understandable: that is, the creation of his new families – three of them – and his new children, and his many projects that were dreamed of and then abandoned, while others were accomplished, in frenetic activity that from the age of fifty onward was characteristic of him, up until the time of his death.

Louis Kahn's creativity passes through continual progressions and reparations, but also through repetitions, and it needs new objects, new investments, new ideas, even if they are unsaturated ones. The son develops a creativity that is the product of a process of working through and of reparation of the internal loved-and-lost object, as well as of the integration of unconscious elements that inhabit his mental life – ones that translate into the construction of a harmonious, enjoyable object that in the end is beautiful.

On a theoretical level, in the case of Nathaniel, we are closer to Hanna Segal's (1958) theory of a creativity that is the product of a deep dialectical exchange between destructive and reparative fantasies, and of the compensatory role of harmony and beauty. In the case of Louis, alongside the reparative mechanisms, there is a powerful emergence of the search for new ideas and the capacity to confront what is unknown and unsaturated. In both father and son, a propelling aspect seems to be the search for psychic truth.

The Fisher House and the reunited family

Nathaniel's trip through the past is made up of stops in front of his father's works and at the locations of the buildings his father designed but never realized.[8] He also pauses before the suffering faces of the women who still cry at the betrayal by the man they loved, and of the friends who pay him homage, moved because of the great gift that they received from him, who also cry when meeting the son for the first time. One of these friends is Robert

Broudrey, who sails his "Symphony Boat," the floating concert hall that Louis built for him, which he had designed one evening in a game with his son: the peculiar ship, the cookie ship, the sausage ship! The "Symphony Boat" still resounds with music, sailing the ocean at sunset, flaming red – perhaps a revisited, sublimated memory of the scorching ember that burned the face of the child Louis?

It is necessary to spend some time with the women whom Nathaniel meets and films, and with their tears: Louis's public wife, Esther, unaware of the existence of the other two women; and his second companion, Anne, who still cries with disappointment for the loss she suffered, but who seems to have reconciled herself with both Kahn's professional stature and his human weaknesses. Finally there is Nathaniel's mother, the most difficult meeting for him; she continues to deny evidence of the betrayal of her/their expectations, and still believes that Louis had no documents with him at the time of his death because he had erased his old identity in order to go and live with them, as he had promised.

Still present between this woman and her son is a knot of unresolved mourning for the man who never re-joined them, but also the effect of a bond of love so tenacious as to make the mother remain faithful to the memory of the only man she had loved. Nathaniel searches for an exit from his mother's blocked mourning and from the possible fossilization of his father's memory; he is almost "obligated" to bring to a conclusion the task of working through in order to find his own truth and creativity.

If on the paternal side the son was able to revisit the father's giant body of work, on the maternal side, he seems in the film to collide with an insurmountable "conviction," as sturdy as the rock on which the mother went to live, isolated within her memories. Perhaps it was that obstinate love, however, that allowed the son to continue to try to understand, and, in that never-completed search, to find something similar to a "father in mother" (Ogden, 1994), a paternal object, a structuring part of the complexity of the ego, rediscovered through the loved "architecture" object, which established their union and made it "dreamable" for the son.

Nathaniel daydreams, in order to re-create the dream that his parents lived together and that he has united them in the love that gave him life. His parents' meeting point can thus be found in their common passion, in the idea of architecture as a continual search, never saturated – an architecture that doesn't exist if not in the works in which one expresses oneself, as his father used to say, and that each person must rediscover in himself, tolerating doubts and the complexity of endless searching.

In their excellent work, Chinaglia and Cornoldi (2008) write:

> The director must not, then, divide the mother with the father, since in fact the mother remained alone, all for him, and did not love other men. The anxiety of the oedipal triangle could thus become a liberation from

> the 'dilemma' and be transformed in 'complexity': the supporting pillar of a healthy narcissism and of creative activity.
>
> (Chinaglia and Cornoldi, 2008)

Louis Kahn accumulated buildings, projects, commissions, romantic relationships, and children in a never-ending race, interrupted only by death, and perhaps just before by the mysterious deletions in his own identity documents.

From the mass of material accumulated by the father, the son sets out on the route of reconstruction and of memory, gathering in his paternal heritage and making it his own. Nathaniel takes on the task of putting people back into contact with each other, of reconnecting affects and fragmented stories, of "acquainting" a family of children who can finally be together, and chooses as the meeting place the beautiful Fisher house, constructed by his father. There Esther's daughter, Sue Ann, a neurologist and a flautist; Anne's daughter Alexandra, an art historian, and Nathaniel meet and ask themselves whether they are a family, without being able to give an answer but neither avoiding the question, together appreciating an environment bequeathed to them by their father.

Louis has constructed a "place" – not only a physical one – in which one can achieve the integration that for him has been impossible, but which he has laid the bases for so that others can bring the work to completion.

Mourning always leaves behind some unsaturated elements, unresolved ones, and much time is needed – sometimes more than a generation – in order to bring it to a close. The working through of mourning also means, perhaps, tolerating that the task may never be completely finished, and that what is important is to leave for others "good materials so that they can continue to create."

Bangladesh: The conclusion of the trip

Louis Kahn travelled and built in various countries. The last sequence of the film was shot in India. "For a moment I returned to being a child," says Nathaniel on arriving in India – perhaps because only a child can truly understand that country, with its strong colours, the expression of joy, as his father had written to him on a postcard. Or perhaps because only there can Nathaniel reclaim the eyes of a child in love with his great father, and only there can he comprehend the eyes of the child/father Louis who sees Bangladesh and bestows a future on it.

In fact, there is a child in front of the parliament building, a building constructed by workers hired by Louis – workers who transported sacks of cement on their heads, as it was done a hundred years ago. In that sequence, the crowded spaces and the empty ones between the buildings are reconnected in the son's imagery. He discovers in himself and represents for us viewers a harmony based on the composition of massive, monolithic Euclidean forms, and of basic geometrical figures – circle, square, triangle – and the strength of simple materials, bare bricks or concrete, which leave transparent the way in which they were assembled revealing both weight-bearing and secondary elements. All are founded on the natural elements of light, water, sky, and air – and all this combines to give Louis Kahn's architecture a unique thickness of monumentality "outside of time."

The building is so improbable in such a poor country, one so far from democracy, but it was considered so monumental and timeless that it escaped bombing during the Indo-Pakistani War. That would certainly have flattered its creator, who would have seen the realization of his idea of an architecture that endures and that, with the passage of time, acquires in monumentality "its original nature of only form and only material" (Chinaglia and Cornoldi, 2007, p. 21).

Nathaniel's trip ends in front of the building that he has chosen as the key to his interior journey. That place seems to represent a paradox for him, the most creative act and at the same time the one that destroyed his father, who died immediately on his return from Bangladesh, most likely stricken by a heart attack. For Nathaniel it seems to coincide with the most arduous point of his journey.

When he confesses his uncertainty – exhausted by all the work he has undertaken on this esoteric trip, both inside and outside himself (for he will dedicate at most ten minutes of his short film to this building), it will be the architect Shamsul Wares, his interlocutor, who will now take upon himself the pain and the waste that would be involved in abandoning the work now; it will be the other who keeps alive the desire to understand and to bring to conclusion the task of documenting the story of his rediscovery of his father. The reaction of the architect, wounded, showing authentic pain in the face of this tired son, trying to understand and to forgive, is one of most moving moments of the film.

For those who do the work of a psychoanalyst, this sequence evokes moments in which we stagger, we totter, and we must fight to keep alive the analytic couple's desire to bring the journey to an end, and not to waste, in a moment of destructive discouragement, the hours of patient and silent searching. The interlocutor's reproof, the tears of pain and anger that filled him and reddened his eyes, restore Nathaniel's desire to conclude the work and his interior journey.

The dream of democracy that Louis Kahn bequeathed to Pakistan, and that perhaps cost him his life, becomes so palpable that it quenches the son's momentary indifference, his rebellion against the fate of having had a fugitive father. His estrangement subsides in contemplating this monument to democracy that perhaps bestows on him, too – the abandoned son – a democracy and a new tolerance in the relationship with his own affects, with his newfound sisters, and with his mother.

Conclusion

In concluding, I will return to the remark that I cited earlier: if the basic material is good and well assembled, there will be a marvellous ruin, and there will thus be a continuity of the transmission of knowledge between father and sons, between great masters and students. This remark contains the love that Louis Kahn, father and architect, had for teaching, for history, for natural, weather-resistant materials – so loved by him that he had theorized the use of perishable materials, ones that would be capable, however, of preserving the impression of the grandeur of something major, of something that would leave a mark.

Thus, Nathaniel's homage to his father is an homage to the grandeur "of a good product without an expiration date," which does not spoil because it is the fruit of an authentic and basic desire to give order and form to things in his career as an architect – and in being a man.

Now that he has found "my architect" of the film's title, one might ask which father Nathaniel Kahn has found. Certainly, in the open and unsaturated spaces between his buildings, between the powerful blocks of his works, each one complete in itself, on the water and in the light that floods the interiors, Nathaniel has discovered an evocative capacity, imaginative and fantastic, which has a paternal flavour and scent.

Which father could rediscover a son accustomed to nocturnal disappearances and sudden reappearances, seduced by extraordinary paternal creativity – a son who felt himself loved, thought about, appreciated, and who was then suddenly abandoned, without explanation, having colluded with maternal denial in the form of a belief that the father was going to live with them?

Not having been overwhelmed by the annihilating anger of having been abandoned without explanation, maintaining a space in which he could put himself in contact with his father and thus save his imaginative capacity, is the encouraging message of this interior journey aimed at the search for the director's affective roots. Nathaniel's creativity turns out to be born not of the complex and contradictory parts of a personality that is instinctively more uninhibited than his father's might have been; it is rather the result of the work of one who patiently observes and "assembles," piece by piece, the sparse fragments left in disorder by the hurried, "maniacal" nature of a genius father.

In the creativity of both of them – and perhaps in creativity in general – there is a leftover portion that remains unexplored, unexplorable, a "mystery" that continues to fascinate us, that we grab hold of and perhaps also penetrate when we let ourselves be invaded by the "beauty" of a work, one that every time makes us feel ourselves to be human beings vibrant with affects.

In more strictly analytic terms, we could invoke with Freud the inexorable and varied push of affects in search of representation, which the two artists, father and son, permit us to live in all their regenerating power.

The work of mourning, the activity of symbolization, and the birth of a representative capacity are connected and interwoven in the most elementary forms of creativity, just as in those that are artistically higher and more complex, like psychic instruments that are activated in order to learn and tolerate the absence or loss of the object.

When and where it is possible to recuperate a representation capable of surviving the absence of the lost object, a potentially creative psychic space is born there, a space that can be revitalized and rendered fertile.

All translations from the Italian by Gina Atkinson.

Notes

1 A previous version of this chapter was published in *Psychoanalytic Quarterly* (2014), 83(2): 441–464.

2 Examples of works of this type are *Un'ora sola ti vorrei* [I would want you for only an hour] (2000), a film by Alina Marazzi, and *Boogie Woogie Daddy* (2003), a film by the Swedish director Erik Bafving. The first of these is a moving and evocative example of the effort of memory to reconstruct/construct an emotional retrospective journey in search of a connection with a mother who committed suicide, lost at a very young age. The director draws inspiration from the 8mm films made by her grandfather, the publisher Ulrico Hoepli, during family holidays and vacations. In *Boogie Woogie Daddy*, Erik Bafving, sets up his short subject by drawing on the numerous photographs left behind by his father, a silent and depressed man who ultimately committed suicide. The quick flashes that record brief moments of family life, in the sad sequence of images assembled by the son make possible a difficult reconstruction and ultimately some measure of consolation for such a dramatic loss. In 2004, on the occasion of the third European Psychoanalytic Film Festival in London, a panel entitled "Sons and Parents" was organized, in which these two films were presented and discussed.

3 The topic of the interaction between art, mourning, and consolation was discussed in an illuminating article by Alexander Stein (2006).

4 This structure, begun in 1963, would be completed posthumously in 1983, nine years after the death of its creator.

5 Philip Johnson is considered the greatest senior architect of the 1900s, the creator of, among other works, the Glass House that appears in this documentary. Vincent Scully is the principal historian of architecture in the United States and bears credit for having launched Kahn's career. I.M. Pei created the pyramid at the Louvre and the National Gallery in Washington, while Frank Gehry is another great contemporary architect.

6 Louis Kahn (1901–1974) was also an excellent artist and a creative virtuoso in music (he was also a composer), and he gained attention beginning in his early years at school for his talent in drawing, obtaining scholarships with which he financed his scholastic career. In fact, his academic performance was not outstanding; he often appeared distracted in the opinion of his teachers, lost in fantasizing and in drawings, perhaps bored by the curriculum. Initially, he undertook artistic studies in the city of Philadelphia, and then, in 1924, obtained a degree in architecture at the University of Pennsylvania. Throughout his life, Louis Kahn never abandoned the teaching he began in 1948 at Yale University and later continued at the University of Pennsylvania, where he remained until his death. He also taught in Europe for some time, leaving an indelible mark on young European architects who experienced the influence of his genius.

7 Matters of image, and of formal and abstract technological experimentation, predominate in functionalism. In modernism, space, light, furnishings, and sensoriality predominate. In the former, aesthetic concerns are foremost; in the latter, those of well-being and functionality.
8 Among these unrealized projects are the Palazzo dei Congressi of Venice (1968–73) and the hotel on Government Hill in Jerusalem (1971–73).

References

Aberbach, David. 1989. "Creativity and the Survivor: The Struggle for Mastery." *International Review of Psycho-Analysis* 16: 273–286.

Algini, Maria Luisa. 2009. "'Elaborare il lutto': Alle strette con Freud." *Rivista di Psicoanalisi* LV(3): 705–724.

Augé, Marc. 2005. *Nonluoghi. Introduzione a un'antropologia della surmodernità.* Milan: Eléuthera.

Bafving, Erik. (dir.) *Boogie Woogie Daddy.* 2002. Sweden: WG Film. Film.

Bernhard, Thomas. 1983. *Il soccombente.* Rome: Adelphi Editore.

Braghieri, Nicola. 2005. *Buoni edifici, meravigliose rovine.* Milan: Giangiacomo Feltrinelli Editore.

Capuano, Marta. 2006. "Introduzione. Louis Kahn: My architect. Un percorso alla ricerca dei uno dei padri dell'architettura moderna." *Architettonicamente Rivista di architettura. Numero speciale 7.* Edizioni ETS.

Chinaglia, Adriano and Alessandra Cornoldi. 2007. "Architettura e Psicoanalisi. Nathaniel Kahn e la Ricerca del Padre." In *La vitalità degli oggetti: esplorazioni attorno al pensiero di C. Bollas.* Rome: Borla.

Freud, Sigmund. 1915. "On Transience." *Standard Edition, Vol. 14.* London: Hogarth Press, pp. 303–307.

Kahn, Louis. 2006. "Conversazioni con gli Studenti." In Marta Capuano (ed.), *My Architect. Un Percorso alla Ricerca di Uno dei Padri dell'Architettura Moderna. Architettonicamente. Rivista di architettura. Numero speciale/7.* Pisa: Edizioni ETS.

Kahn, Louis. 2002. "Louis I. Kahn Talks." In Maria Bonaiti (ed.) *Architettura E'.* Milan: Electa.

Kahn, Nathaniel. (dir.) *My Architect.* 2004. USA: Louis Kahn Project Inc. Film.

Marazzi, Alina. (dir.) *Un'ora sola ti vorrei.* 2002. Italy: Venerdì, Bartlebyfilm, RTSI, TELE+. Film.

Ogden, Thomas H. 1994. *Subjects of Analysis.* London: Karnac.

Ogden, Thomas H. 2004. "This Art of Psychoanalysis." *International Journal of Psychoanalysis* 85: 857–877.

Racalbuto, Agostino. 1994. *Tra il Fare e il Dire.* Milan: Raffaello Cortina Editore.

Racalbuto, Agostino. 2001. "Saxa Loquuntur!" In A. Racalbuto, M. La Scala and M.V. Costantini (eds), *La Nascita della Rappresentazione fra Lutto e Nostalgia.* Rome: Borla.

Segal, Hanna. 1958. "Fear of death – Notes on the Analysis of an Old Man." *International Journal of Psychoanalysis* 39: 178–181.

Stein, Alexander. 2006. "Music, Mourning, and Consolation." *Journal of the American Psychoanalytic Association,* 52: 787–811, translated as "Musica, Lutto e consolazione." *Rivista italiana di Psicoanalisi* LII: 783–812.

Winnicott, Donald W. 1992. *Through Paediatrics to Psychoanalysis: Collected Papers*: London: Institute of Psychoanalysis and Karnac Books.

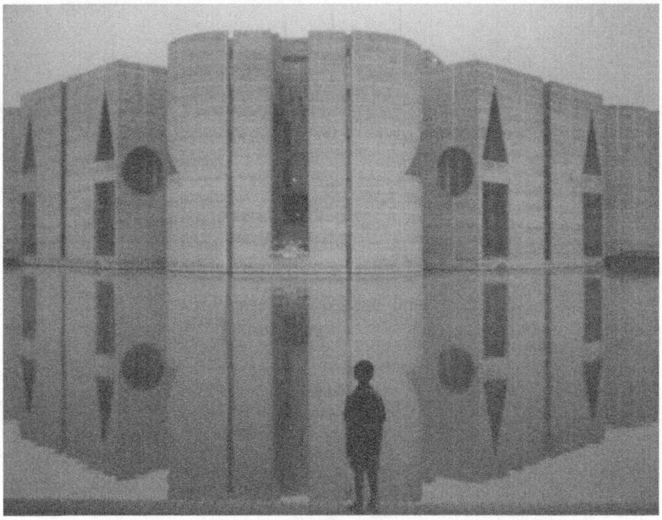

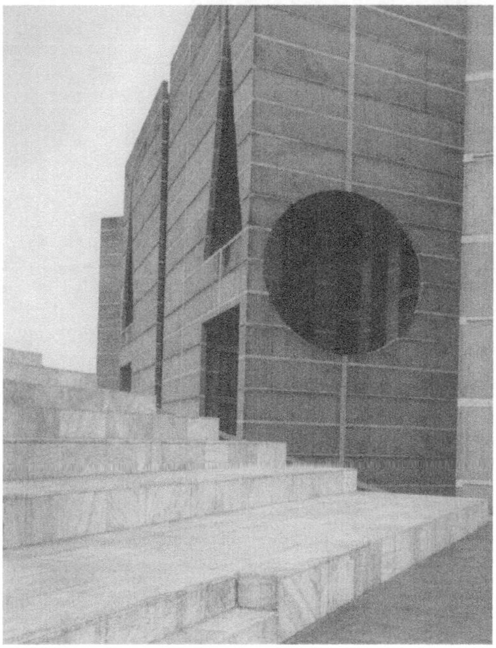

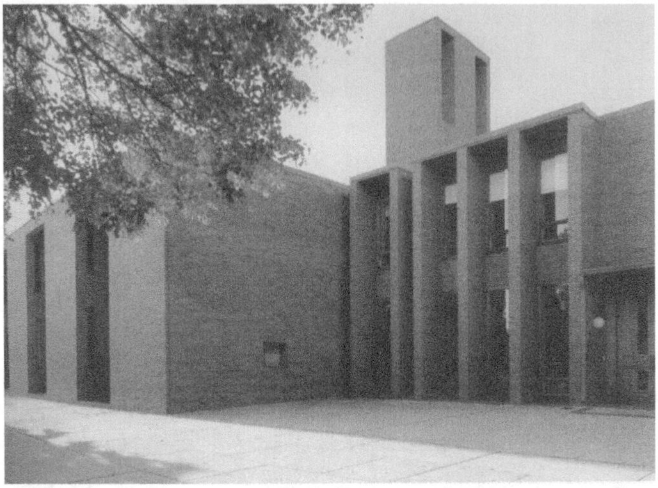

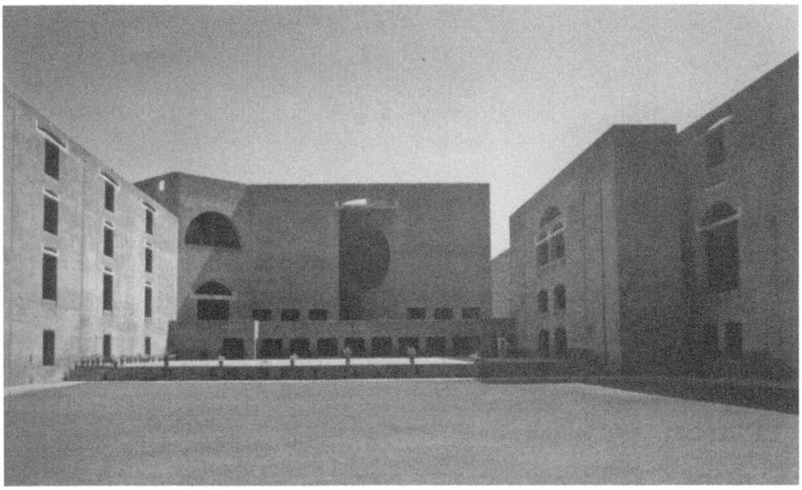

Chapter 5

Feminine representations on the screen

Brodeuses by Éléonore Faucher[1]

A woman's gaze on a woman's body

Brodeuses [Sequins], the first film of the scriptwriter and director Éléonore Faucher (2004), was nominated for a César award in 2005. Recounted from a feminine viewpoint, the film explores both the physical and psychic changes of a woman during her first pregnancy.

The extraordinary understanding between the actors (Ariane Ascaride and Lola Naymark) along with the director's attention to the characters' physical expressions create perceptive, affective and memorable conditions that guide us towards a truth which is waiting to be discovered, a truth whose meaning exists beyond the events of this story, which is focused on the emotions and deeper values of everyday life.

Claire (Lola Naymark), a beautiful red-headed girl, is faced with an age-old dilemma, something is happening inside of her; she is experiencing an event which is as old as the hills we see in the first scenes of the film: an unwanted teenage pregnancy.

We soon realize that Claire is living in two different realities: on the one hand, the weight of her daily struggle for survival; on the other, a separate, intimate reality marked by her new, burgeoning secret, but also by soft rabbit skins which she barters for cabbages stolen from her parents' field and which she adorns with sequins and glitter: a world of bright embroidery where her artistic skills are put to the test. Her pregnancy gets in the way of these two worlds and biological time is pressing on her for a choice she is not prepared to take.

She goes to a pregnancy advisory centre: the female doctor appreciates the girl's difficulties in dealing with the situation and that she attempts to deny its evidence. The doctor insists that it is be important to know what stage of pregnancy Claire is in and she mentions the possibility of giving birth to her child anonymously. Claire seems to be tempted by this option, because it is very difficult for her to think about the baby now, she is still too concerned about her body image which is being reshaped by pregnancy. She is ashamed of it, she fears she might become the object of disapproving looks, she wants to give birth to her baby away from home.

The doctor is the first adult woman who understands what Claire's physical and psychological conditions really are. She keeps a professional distance, but she is competent and, little by little, she overcomes the girl's opposition. She persuades the girl to have an ultrasound scan and she invites her to look at the foetus as it moves inside her: Claire, however, averts her eyes, she only fleetingly looks at her swollen belly which she cannot yet recognize, she does not want to see, she does not even want to know the baby's sex: yet she is clearly upset, she is moved. Deep inside, something has been set into motion: she does not deny any longer what she is actually experiencing. She then asks the doctor to write the baby's sex on a piece of paper which she will hide – without reading it – in a place no one else knows: a cassette player, an object symbolizing her adolescence.

The gaze of the first woman to see her pregnant state has forced her to accept the evidence of her four-to-five-month expectant belly. A concerned, benevolent, maternal gaze helps her at least to look at the baby that is growing inside her: thanks to a first, empathic contact between the doctor and herself, Claire can look with new eyes at the foetus she is carrying in her womb.

A statement which would sound familiar to any analyst: psychic wounds can be healed only through an in-depth process which unwinds the tangled web of associations and reconstructions.

Some thoughts on female psychosexual development

When Freud (1923) writes that the Ego is first and foremost a body ego, he refers to the psychic representation of an image or body scheme, which is already separated from the maternal body and from the outside world. From the very beginning, the theme of the relationship between mind and body is interwoven with anxiety; but in 1926, writing "Inhibition, Symptoms and Anxiety", Freud introduces a developmental concept of anxiety by describing the specific dangers that occur during different phases of development – beginning with separation anxiety from the maternal object which he believes serves as the prototype to all the successive ones.

Freud differentiates male anxiety from female anxiety. He believes that male anxiety is linked to the fear of castration while the female's is linked to the little girl's danger of the loss of the love of the object, which Freud believes stems from separation from the primary (maternal) object.

The maternal function is referred to as the primary protective shield (Freud, 1926), an anti-stimulus barrier. Authors like Winnicott (1992) and Bion (1962), by studying the early stages of development and by introducing the concepts of holding function and reverie, have reached a more complete understanding of the significance of the mother's affective relationship with the infant's body. These characteristics of the relationship with the mother allow the child to perceive the boundaries of his/her own body, to invest in him/herself, in his/her own functions and erogenous zones – thus determining their future development.

The little girl's psychosexual development and the definition of the boundaries of her body are made more complex by the need to identify herself while also needing to disidentify herself from her mother/primary object; and by the difficulty of differentiating her own body from the maternal body, which was her first object of investment.

In a recent book on gender identity, Doris Bernstein (1993), among others, states that the girl's development, her anxieties and psychic fantasies must be investigated in relation to the body and to its changes as the girl becomes a woman, and to the difficulties of making definite mental representations of it in relation to the ups and downs of the daughter's separation from the mother.

Consequently, every time a new developmental phase occurs for the girl and her body undergoes deep changes, as in adolescence or in pregnancy,[2] given that the bond with the mother has not yet been entirely resolved, separation anxieties return creating conflict in the girl's acceptance of her own "new" sexually adult body. This will affect how and when the oedipal dynamics will be faced and when the differentiation and the separation from the body of the parent of the same sex are able to consolidate itself. It will also affect when reality-testing replaces infantile omnipotence (Laufer, 2006). Turning to her mother for help in getting through the developmental stages, the daughter finds herself having to face the anxiety, which stems from this very conflict. On one hand the girl needs to identify with the mother, it is this mature type of identification that the young girl needs to reinforce, yet at the same time there is a regressive counter-tendency to return to being "mummy's little girl", which is reactivated just at the point when more developed identifications are taking place. In becoming a woman and a mother, the girl's body becomes a woman's body, the object of men's desires. The girl has to therefore confront herself again with her mother who is now an oedipal rival, and experience the anxieties caused by the separation-individuation from that maternal body which at the beginning of life was "everything". Now, instead she has to learn to feel her body as similar to her mother's, but yet distinct and separate.

Adolescence and pregnancy

The extensive and deep physical and mental transformations of pregnancy produce a real re-organization between the balance of narcissistic and object investments. Therefore pregnancy can represent a moment of crisis which can bring forth again intense separation anxieties: on the one hand it offers the opportunity to achieve a new level of self-organization, on the other, it is open to a possible involution (Bibring et al., 1961). Some authors consider it the last step of the separation-individuation process from the mother (Pines, 1982).

A young pregnant woman has to change her relationship with herself in order to identify with the role of her mother. In this situation it is possible that old defences that were utilized during developmental crisis in relationship to one's own body are then reactivated. The body has to become the object of a new libidinal narcissistic investment, which helps the young girl negotiate the possession of a female body and to become a mother who is able to feel pleasure from her baby's body. If not, she may become vulnerable to self-destructive impulses – she may have an abortion or decide not to keep her own baby. According to Egle Laufer (1982), becoming a mother involves the loss of the libidinal bond with the girl's own mother and her body; a strong residual attachment to the maternal body is therefore an obstacle to the elaboration of the mourning of this loss.

An undesired pregnancy

The plot of the movie is based on the encounter between Claire (Lola Naymark) and Mme Mélikian (Ariane Ascaride): the girl, Claire, is pregnant, the woman, Mme Mélikian, has recently lost her only son in an accident. They meet because of their common interest in embroidery, this meeting will change their lives.

Claire denies the evidence of her pregnancy, even in front of the ultrasound scan, and when the woman doctor invites her to watch the foetus as it moves inside her, she averts her eyes. It is difficult for her to accept the reality of her rapidly changing body, so she tries to conceal it by adding layers of clothing; she feels ashamed and fears the disapproving glances of others.

Shame, fear and denial are her present feelings. When her colleagues unkindly point out that she is putting on weight, Claire employs a terrible lie in self-defence. She says she is ill and must have cortisone and chemotherapy treatment, which bloats her and causes hair-loss. To persuade them of this, she tears out a clump of hair in front of them.

This terrible lie springs from her deep ambivalence, the struggle between love and hate, libido and thanatos, which is taking place inside her, in her belly and in her mind, where an "object" is growing, which she has yet to recognize as part of herself and has yet to invest with libido.

For the moment, destructiveness and persecutory feelings prevail.

At night, she dreams her head is resting in a woman's lap; the red-haired woman (her mother) strokes her hair and gently pulls out long locks. The scene, which with its bluish-leaden colouring is reminiscent of certain works of sixteenth- and seventeenth-century northern European painting, betrays her emotional freezing and the death anxiety, which follows her angry outburst against herself in front of her colleagues. The sweetly maternal gesture is turned into horror at the sight of her hair, the symbol of beauty (the girl's most important female attribute), falling lifeless in a *fatal transmission* from mother to daughter, where instead, warmth and affection should flow.

The representation of the dreamlike image reveals the dark/unresolved side of the mother/daughter relationship, in which envy, destructiveness, jealousy and castration are still woven together in a malicious way and come back to the surface at this key moment of Claire's psychosexual development.

Pregnancy appears here because of Claire's youth and the situation in which she finds herself as a *turning point*, which reactivates ancient narcissistic wounds. Denying the reality of the changes which are happening to her body, Claire temporarily denies the very reality of the baby which has yet to be born – in fact, she wants to have the baby anonymously. In other words, she wants to give the baby away, get rid of it.

A freezing mother's gaze

During adolescence girls have the task of modifying their relationship with their bodies, from that of a prepubescent girl to that of a sexually active adult woman.

Claire finds herself pregnant, while she is probably still dealing with the great physical transformations of adolescence. Her pregnancy, therefore, appears to her to be the result of a mechanical accident: a condom too full of air, which "burst inside her" while she was having sex, not with a boy she loves and desires, but with a married man. Having lost the physical integrity of her childhood and adolescence, she now experiences her body as a bruised and alien cavity, in which things she is ashamed of are taking place; it is an unknown body without the reparation of a sufficiently gratifying mother's glance (Winnicott, 1992).[3]

It seems there is an unbridgeable gap between her present life and her abruptly ended adolescence, between her job in the supermarket (where she feels the gaze of the enquiring eyes of her colleagues, or by the unfriendly, greedy glance of the young man in the butchery department whom we later discover is the baby's father) and her separate, private reality.

Her deep ambivalence seems generated also by her need to defend a potentially creative yet secret dimension (another secret she cannot confess to anyone), the soft rabbit skins she has bartered for the cabbages stolen from her parents' field. She adorns the pelts with sequins and glitter and in this regressive dimension of play, seems to be able once more to find a sense of narcissistic integrity, which has been put into doubt by the pregnancy.[4]

The importance the film gives to the eyes, the glances, and the sequins that glitter, appears as a poetic translation of Claire's need to re-establish a good-enough relation with her primary maternal object/vital nucleus of her Self. That relationship is based on mirroring (Winnicott, 1967) between the maternal look and the infant's response: from that mirroring the baby creates its mother in the moment in which it creates itself and its world, to make it a safe place for itself.

More recently Florence Guignard (2010) has described the need of a girl to "represent the invisible". This is a complex work of representation of the inner world, begun during puberty and should, ideally, be finished with the birth of the first child. The process is initiated by something concrete – the developing foetus – pushing for representation for the necessity of the psyche to take possession of one's own inner Self. This too is part of the conclusion at the drive level of the working-through of the feminine identification, in particular of the transformation from a narcissistic identification to the secondary one.

From mother to daughter

Claire's story and the elaboration which her pregnancy brings her to, is interwoven with the different types of mourning the other characters, Guillaume and Mme Mélikian, have endured.

Guillaume is her best friend Lucille's brother. His face is scarred by a recent injury. With just a few telling images, we discover another drama, which interweaves with Claire's: a motorcycle accident, the violent death of a young man, Isham, and his mother's (Mme Mélikian) desperation.

In the background, we hear the irritating, shrew-like voice of Guillaume's mother, who is beating, skinning and cutting with brutal indifference the live eel her son has caught. It is not difficult to imagine that this woman treats all that pulses with life and emotions in the same way, including her husband's virility and authority. Indeed, her husband is little more than a big baby reduced to dealing with insignificant details, such as opening walnuts without breaking them and then admiring them in an infantile manner, in partial reparation of the castration he has undergone in his relations with his wife. Just as Claire's mother has never noticed her daughter's pregnancy and has probably insufficiently noticed her needs, Lucille's mother cannot see the situation before her very eyes: the anxiety of the adolescent Claire left by adults to make enormous decisions by herself, the wounded soul and feelings of guilt which threaten to overwhelm her own son, Guillaume, who has now left his job and wants to live by hunting and catching fish. He too, is like Claire, in search of a primitive regressive dimension.

Claire's gift for embroidery is seen only as a practical opportunity, so Lucille's mother suggests that she ask Mme Mélikian, an expert embroiderer, about becoming her assistant as a replacement for her deceased son. Lucille's mother, like Claire's and other minor female figures in the film (the baker, for example) seem to reproduce models of identification with women who reduce existence to a series of hard and repetitive daily chores through which control and apparent security is assured. Their worlds revolve around food and domestic work; they thus devitalize the affective dimension and creativity. Women like these demean the male, defrauding him of his virile and paternal function, while maintaining a female universe which is in danger of depriving even biological creativity of its joy. Indeed, Claire has great difficulty in finding within herself the joy of becoming a mother, since she has probably never seen that joy reflected in her mother's eyes or, if so, only fleetingly. She seems to find it in the transferred splendour of the sequins and shiny paillettes of her embroidery.

Pregnancy and working through

The contact with what is left of her dreams of embroidery, and with the sorrow on the face of Guillaume, seems to give Claire the stimulus to begin working through her own mourning for what she has lost. She leaves work in the supermarket to enact her plan to become an embroiderer; Claire gathers up her best embroideries, hides her splendid hair in a headscarf that completely covers her head – a sign of her depressive capacity to place herself under the authority of a competent adult – and rings Mme Mélikian's doorbell.

This is the start of a slow but delicate interweaving of the working through of two bereavements (perhaps even three, if we include that of Guillaume), in an ideal process of "female-style" reparation. Both the protagonists are in the throes of mourning, which affect their femininity; both are fascinated by sequins and needlework and are united by their creativity and passion for embroidery.[5]

Together, set in motion by recent bereavements, each reactivates old deep wounds. One has undergone object loss – the death of her son; the other has endured a narcissistic loss. However, as Freud (1915) reminds us: every loss is always narcissistic. As these two women continue to meet, Claire's baby expects increasingly becomes an emotionally invested object, while Mme Mélikian recovers part of herself which has been obscured by the shadow of the object, her lost son. Her workshop has for Claire all the charm of an enchanted world, a mother's womb, so bright she can finally reflect herself in it.

As in the best fairy tales, it is no easy task to enter the desired place; first you must undergo a test, that is to learn "to go deeper" to produce something lasting. The two women initiate a co-production, a sort of alliance which is concrete and symbolic, external and internal: Claire listens and learns, with the confidence of someone who knows they have found what they were looking for; the adult understands more than she then is able to say on Claire's pregnancy. Claire has re-awakened in her the desire for life, but she is still deeply wounded in her femininity and motherhood.

The light of the maternal gaze

Claire and Mme Mélikian exchange glances in which they transmit the intuition of a mutual need and the basic desire that attracts one to the other. The girl needs to be observed and seen by a woman/mother in order to grow up and become in her turn a mother capable of loving. The middle-aged woman needs the life, which Claire has within her, to fill her inner emptiness, which is in danger of destroying her identity and life itself. Both have a female wound to heal, the glimmering of a desire to find again the beauty and splendour of a mother's glance when her eyes sparkle with joy or shine with love and emotion for her child. One woman runs the risk of not seeing the baby she is about to bear, the other cannot see her child because he is lost to her.

The sequins and shiny buttons which Claire attaches to her embroidery, expertly sewing them on to the veils and precious material, working side by side with Mme Mélikian, represent the sublimated aspect of the maternal look which she gradually begins to feel upon herself and which the older woman little by little begins to cast on her. For Claire, this means being able to reclaim her body, so changed by pregnancy, acknowledging the change and thus making mental space for the baby inside her. At first an internal persecutory object, the baby can now become part of her self, a libidinally invested object.

Because of a failure in the relationship with the primary object and therefore the lack of the mother's look in which to reflect herself, she experienced the man's penis in her sexual encounter as a partial object charged with unresolved oedipal conflicts. Claire has, in fact, "stolen" it by engaging in a secret affair with a married man, himself a father. Likewise, her creativity seems to be linked to theft (stealing cabbages from her parents). Therefore, the sexual act which made her pregnant had no reparative effect, but only highlights the partial failure of her relationship with the maternal primary object (Rupprecht-Shampera, 1997).

In symbolic terms, the paternal penis was unable to perform its structuring function as a "bridge" (Freud, 1920) between the child's maternal world, which is merged and concrete, and the paternal one, which is symbolic and separate. Instead, it has become the bearer of an identity crisis, brought on by her unwanted pregnancy, and the baby – equated with the penis – is in danger of undergoing the same fate and therefore of being rejected.

Pregnancy thus becomes the moment of crisis in Claire's deficient affective development. To the baby growing inside her, she cannot give what she has insufficiently received from her own mother. This is why Claire hides, covers herself up and plans to give away the baby as soon as it is born, as if it were a debased object, nameless, and part of a chain of an anonymous evacuative transmission.

Both women need to regress benignly to a maternal, female world, intended here as a dyadic relationship from which males are temporarily shut out – since males come within a paternal code, which is triadic and tends towards separation.

The dyadic relationship of the two women recalls certain analyses, which must proceed at length without interpretations that denote separateness, immersion in silence or hushed words, with fleeting glances exchanged at the beginning and end of the session. In such moments, one has the impression of tapestry weaving, a subtle embroidery which might be torn asunder by poorly timed interpretations.

There is a beautiful scene in which the two women work in silence on the great embroidery; one is expertly skilled, the other willing and helpful. Both are joyful. As they work, like the fabric in their hands, the story of their inner life is enriched and repaired, under the protection of a male figure, which they have found again, at least in an ideal sense, in the guise of Lacroix, the famous designer who has commissioned the precious embroidery.

That we are witnessing a trauma of womanhood which can only be worked through in a "female" dimension is confirmed by the fact that the male characters are, for the most part, insignificant to the plot. The butcher who got Claire pregnant is predatory and malicious; when faced with the news of her pregnancy, he merely suggests an evacuatory solution, offering money for an abortion. Claire's friend's father is reduced to childishness. Guillaume is depressed and wounded, while others are distant or idealized like the designer, Lacroix, who might even be the secret father of Mme Mélikian's dead son.

In the silence of the workshop where all that can be heard is the sound of a sewing machine, symbolising the work which brings them together, the two women work through their respective losses, each mirroring the other. In a continuous interweaving, each put something of herself into the other. By observing and discovering the elegance and femininity of the other woman, Claire is again placed in touch with herself, her body and the child she is carrying. A timid dialogue starts up between the two women, an exchange of memories and confessions; a mother-daughter dialogue, one might say.

Deep empathic understanding develops between the two women: it is characterized by a short phase of merging and regression in the service of the Ego and fostered by the wish to perform a common task. In fact, Claire wants to learn while Mme Mélikian – in spite of her grief – wants to pass on, the ancient knowledge of embroidery matched with something far more deeply valuable, that is, the ability to let life – not just biological life, but also and foremost psychic and affective life – grow and develop.

While the two women apply themselves to embroidery in attentive, industrious silence – a poetic, metaphorical image for what is going on in the analytic room – benign breaches open up in the Self, as Bolognini (2004a) would have it. Through these breaches, words can have access to parts which could not be reached before, boundary areas where human frailties have signs which cannot still be put into words. In fact, these are mainly sensory areas. In the movie, the act of touching the fabric is charged with primordial meaning through displacement: it is a sort of second skin torn apart by recent traumata.

It is, therefore, at pre-verbal level that reparation is set into motion through the metaphor of embroidery, whereas I believe that the sparkle and the characters' special fascination with sequins and glitter metaphorically remind us of unresolved oedipal aspects which come up again and are finally confronted with, as I will try to explain in the lines that follow.

The two main characters – like an analytic couple working at this level – meet within an intermediate psychic area at the boundary between inner and outer world, where "a healthy, physiological fluctuation between regression and progression, merging and separation, primary and secondary process can be achieved" (Bolognini, 2004a, p. 157). This fluctuation guarantees good-enough psychic functioning and – during analysis – for a good treatment outcome.

As already mentioned, it is a sensory, pre-verbal area which has become porous thanks to the analytic encounter: within this area, "... a two-way passage of undifferentiated elements takes place, reminding of what had happened during the first encounter with the maternal object" (Fonda 2000, p. 6). Fonda defines these areas "limited merging areas", "fusional channels" (ibid., p. 3) where contents flow from the child to the mother and backwards, and in the analytic relationship from the patient to the analyst and backwards. In this way, it is possible to attain a state of "confusion/indistinction nesting affective or traumatic contents which could not be explored before" (ibid., p. 4).

These are areas of the Self where the infant and his/her caregiving object can exceed their boundaries and merge in an undifferentiated condition which allows the infant to experience both the mother's sensory presence as well as her mental functioning, while the mother can get "from within the child" messages and shades of meaning which could not be grasped otherwise.

When analyst and patient reach those areas, the contents they exchange are not necessarily tied to words and interpretation, but rather to the stability of the analytic setting and to the emotional "endurance" of the relationship which contribute to weave anew the primary relational fabric that can potentially be torn apart in time of crisis or after traumatic events.

When an analyst is at work, she/he is in tune with those psychic areas lacking delimitation between inner and outer world, body and mind, me and not-me, where the boundary between intrapsychic and interpsychic is indistinct and continually renegotiated (Bolognini, 2011).

It is in this very dimension that useful elements are conveyed to heal recent and past traumatic wounds, according to the Freudian concept of *Hilflosigkeit* and *Nachträglichkeit*, of the first and second moment of the trauma.

In the whole course of life, these wounds can be active at an unconscious, pre-verbal, pre-symbolic level: they can re-emerge in time of crisis, and pregnancy is a time of crisis in the same way as bereavement. These micro- and macro-traumatic elements undermine the affective-sensory shield allowing for a first, rudimentary integration of the Self to take shape, that is, that very primeval feeling to dwell in a body defined by boundaries which Ogden (1989) called an autistic-contiguous position. While adopting the Kleinian-Bionian model describing the schizo-paranoid and depressive position, he also introduced the autistic-contiguous position, a mode whereby the mind organizes reality through the sensory experiences activated by maternal care. According to Ogden, in order to reach the best psychophysical development it is essential for these three positions to interact so that a human being can establish relationships with others along a continuum spanning from a condition of total absence of boundaries to a condition marked by well-defined boundaries between the Self and the Other.

When two minds at work in the analytic room jointly reach this very level of functioning, they exchange something that can restart mental representation – a function which had come to a halt or else had never been activated – provided that a psyche-soma apparatus is made available to hold the affect.

In the film, the body is massively present: as far as Claire is concerned, it is a body macroscopically reshaped by pregnancy, which has turned her life upside down while reactivating an ancient trauma through a new one. As for Madame Mélikian, it is the body of her dead son Isham, whose unbearable, untimely death secluded her in an autistic withdrawal. Mme Mélikian's attachment to the girl runs the risk of being a denial of the terrible loss she has suffered, replacing her son with Claire and putting herself in the pregnant girl's shoes.

As life gradually begins to pulse in her veins once more, her grief becomes increasingly hard to bear, and it culminates in a suicide attempt. It is Claire who saves her. She cannot allow herself to lose the object she has only just found again, but neither can she agree to be a replacement for another, whose identity goes unrecognized. Claire brings Guillaume, who is responsible for Isham's death, to Mme Mélikian's hospital bed, in order to help her deal with the trauma and grief.

The importance of body language and the working through of the harrowing separation from the body of the loved ones are emphasized throughout the film: Mme Mélikian touches Guillaume with heart-rending nostalgia for the body of her lost son; Claire symbolically re-explores her mother's body by lying on Mme Mélikian's bed and taking in her perfume. She admires the chandelier and shimmering glass of her bedroom, tries out the powder puff and chooses the clothes to take to the hospital. She no longer acts furtively like a thief, but rather like a curious child observing her mother. She dares to look at the "underside" to appreciate the true skill of the embroiderer, and is spellbound by the glistening sequins, as if looking through a child's eyes at the wonderful things which comprise her mother's womb.

The two women become conscious of their need for one another, thus establishing a new continuity across the generations and the transmission of knowledge. Left to her own devices, Claire would probably have made an irremediable choice regarding her baby, while Isham, Mme Mélikian's son, would have died again symbolically in his mother's inner world, if she had missed the opportunity that life has offered her in rediscovering her maternal function.

Now that the deep, basic "feminine wound" has been healed, Claire is able to recover her appetite for life and to reveal that she is with child. She tries with her mother, who once again notices nothing and still cannot see. Claire's grief at her mother's inability to acknowledge her does however, becomes tolerable. She weeps, but dreams she is standing by her mother's side, holding in her arms a toddler, perhaps a younger brother who is no longer seen as a rival, or a son she can take care of. She has achieved separation from her mother, who in the dream is by her side, yet at a slight distance.

She is finally able to approach a man and desire him. She allows Guillaume – himself wounded and depressed, but no longer an unhinged, homicidal motorcyclist – to bend down on the pretext of admiring the embroidery and look at her belly, the most intimate part of her creative nature. She teaches him how to touch her body and give her pleasure, and he accepts the presence of a baby in the body of the woman he desires. She re-establishes in her Self the symbolic link between the man's penis and the baby, thus giving a father to the baby she is carrying.

Her pregnancy is no longer just a biological condition, a matter of feeling full of eggs like the trout which Guillaume threw back into the lake, "I'm full of eggs, too," she said. It is no longer a narcissistic wound which triggers denial and anger against femininity and hatred of males. Reparation enables her to envisage the entry of a third. Claire can also consider the baby's sex and tell Mme Mélikian with a smile that it's a girl, confirmation of her renewed ability to appreciate herself and her femininity.

Conclusion

The path traced by cinema narration is very similar to that which takes place, ideally, in the analyst's office, where therapeutic relations are formed and developed, deep wounds healed and desires and affects set in motion once again. At first, the analytic couple – like the two women in the film – moves in a dimension made up of sometimes lengthy silences, careful not to break the symbiotic fabric which will repair the "splits": the premature separation or unbearable loss.

The film shows the importance of profound, affective interaction, which propels the integrating elements, including those tied to sublimation. The encounter between the two protagonists enables the girl to become more aware of her creative ability and Mme Mélikian to recover her creative vitality, crushed by bereavement.

Both re-explore aspects of their early mental functioning, which are pre-symbolic, close to being sensorial, corporeal. In this they are aided by their embroidery, their love for things that glisten, which lies between them like an intermediate, transitional, pre-symbolic space: they thus repair a basic narcissistic deficiency and each feels again that they are "the light of the other's eyes." Both women rediscover their ability to enjoy the beauty of the object and the self (Meltzer, 1973), each affecting in the other a transformation from negativity towards an area of aesthetic sharing which they had lost in their psychic rebellion against mourning (Freud, 1915).

Hable con Ella by Pedro Almodóvar[6]

Bad news and traditional fairy tales: an introduction

The news has familiarized us with the story of young people in irreversible comas who end up being kept in a state of non-life/non-death by modern medicine. The great emotional impact of these events, in addition to the manipulative and perverse use that the media often makes of them, is ascribable to their exemplary nature. But it is also because similar stories take root in the primordial collective imagination, even in the enchanted world of fairy tales that we have all loved since childhood: we all remember that in "Snow White" and "Sleeping Beauty," young girls in a state of apparent death are awakened by the love of a young prince.

I will not concern myself here with the metaphorical significance of those fairy tales; rather it interests me to emphasize the persistence and re-emergence of the stereotype of masculinity and femininity, that in *Hable con Ella* [Talk to Her], Pedro Almodóvar (2002) takes to extremes to explore its complexity and de-construct it.

Specific analytic themes and questions involving the collective imagination are woven together, as many psychoanalytic studies of the film have emphasized, demonstrating the enormous capacity of the cinema to explore human emotions and affectivity. Almodóvar has achieved a maturity of expression in this film that permits us as viewers to undergo a journey that engenders hope and a sense of friendship and love, passing through psychic areas and characters' dimensions in which unfinished gender identifications and personalities may be comprehended, and even a personality so distant and alien from our usual shared meanings – that is, Benigno's – is no longer simply condemned with a label, because something during our viewing of the film will have profoundly changed. (Sabbadini, 2007).

Reflecting on the theme of gender differences in the analytic relationship leads to the consideration of two extreme conditions: that of violating the boundaries in the male analyst/female patient couple, and that of a regressive push toward fused dynamics and states of undifferentiation when both analyst and patient are women. These two conditions seem to highlight the theme of gender rigidity and, at the opposite end of the spectrum, of gender ambiguity. The latter is often seen as the prerogative of the analyst and the artist, who are sometimes called upon to cross new frontiers in the direction of undifferentiation, in an attempt to decipher the traumatic anxiety that is reactivated in the analytic encounter with emotionality and the unconscious world of another human being, and to allow us to imagine what was previously unimaginable.

The plot

Almodóvar's modern "fairy tale" proposes a version that is rougher than the traditional one.

The journalist Marco, returning from an unhappy love affair with a drug addict and in so much pain that he does not speak, attends to his new lover, the toreador Lydia, a patient who remains in a coma after an accident in the ring. Marco discovers during her recuperation that Lydia betrayed him; she no longer loved him and had returned to her former lover, a toreador himself. Meanwhile, in the same clinic, Marco meets Benigno, a nurse who cares for Alicia, a young ballerina in a coma for four years, after a car accident.

The two men are united in close friendship that leads Marco to stick by Benigno even after the latter is imprisoned for having violated and impregnated Alicia. Benigno ends up killing himself in jail, while Marco, after Lydia's death, may fall in love with Alicia, revived after having given birth to a dead baby.

Although the film's male protagonists follow two different routes, their paths are interwoven: one of the two will succumb after having outlined for the other a sort of extreme limit from which to begin again in re-establishing the conversation about love, and after having gone through territories that extend beyond the unthinkable (the violation of a girl's comatose body, the life that is reborn from an almost-dead body).

Pina Bausch's *Café Muller*

From the beginning we are aware that we will be witnessing a representation, introduced by the ballet *Café Muller* by Pina Bausch: the curtain goes up and two dancers with their eyes closed like sleepwalkers, and with faces of suffering, move in a place that is full of chairs, and a man with a very worried air removes the chairs in front of them so that they will not collide with them.

Two spectators come into the frame. One is Benigno, who spies on Marco, who is crying nearby. The scene rapidly changes and Benigno cares for Alicia, a comatose girl, together with a colleague – washing her inert body, including its intimate parts.

When Benigno dresses Alicia in a white gown, the figure of the immobilized woman in bed and the figures of the ballerinas are linked together in a surprising visual continuity, almost as though to clinch the importance of finding connections, of visual and narrative linking, as if to say that this is a film about broken ties and ties that must be reconnected.

The use of artistic and gender anomalies

As T.S. Eliot (1936), wrote, human beings cannot bear too much reality, and certain truths can be approached only under specific conditions, which art and psychoanalysis permit. As in an analytic process the possibility to explore unknown territory requires a setting, a *mise en abime*, in order to set in motion the capacity for representation.

In the movie, the artistic anomalies – the ballets, the songs, the bullfight, and the silent film – become narrative devices that facilitate the approach toward situations that test the human capacity to tolerate pain and loss. For example, the insertion into the soundtrack of the popular "Cucurucucù Paloma," sung by Caetano Veloso, permits Marco to enter into contact with his pain over the loss of his love and to cry. Lyric and music become a salve for pain, but they also have a holding function that facilitates the metamorphosis of affects. Crying is usually considered a non-masculine characteristic, therefore Marco, who is depicted in the film as the expert on love and women, in comparison with the virginal and ambiguous Benigno, immediately appears less rigid, more flexible, from a gender perspective. Parallel to artistic ones, gender anomalies become a path toward metamorphosis and the possible overcoming of gender stereotypes.

Men on the verge of a nervous breakdown

Almodóvar has represented in his films a feminine universe that is rich in complexity and creativity, energetic and vital, and he has not made a secret of being less inspired by men, whom he has defined as boring. In *Talk to Her*, however, he puts men at the centre of his story, entrusting to men the task of resuming the interrupted affective and loving communication. The dramatic nature of the interruption in communication is represented by the women's comatose state, while the two men cannot detach themselves from the intense need to resume communicating, and the viewer with them. Beginning with the film's title, in fact, the verb "talk" emphasizes the necessity of the verbal connection between human beings. Upon this connection Freud founded his treatment method and the theoretical construction of psychoanalysis; In "Attacks on Linking" (1959), Bion emphasized the creative function of a "path" between two objects.

With the words "to her" in the title, the two objects in question assume, furthermore, a precise gender imprint. This is about the talking of men to women, in order to recover a fruitful bond in the relationship between the "intimate strangers" of the film's final song.

Alongside the men and women, almost between them, carriers as they are of partial identifications, there are figures of ambiguous sexual identity, Benigno and Lydia, but perhaps we would have to say that all four of the film's characters demonstrate that "whatever we may say about the biological certainties of sexuality, gender is an encounter with ambiguity" (Lichtenstein, 2005, p. 909).

In contrast to Almodóvar's other films, in which gender ambiguity is provocatively displayed in the climate of the *movida* of maniacal derision at the rigid and conforming mentality of a Spain only recently emerged from dictatorship,[7] the characters of Benigno and Lydia, in particular, seem to serve the function of portraying bisexual resourcefulness, and they act as intermediaries toward redefining personal identity and romantic life, even though they are themselves condemned to emotional failure. They become a path/bridge toward a new definition of the couple and of a loving relationship. Therefore, in *Talk to Her* the game of multiple gender identity is recast in the more complex game of human emotionality, with the painful price of separation and loss no longer denied.

Even the theme of death which in Almodóvar's early films appeared in the form of suicide and murder, is here accidental, determined by chance (Alicia's accident), or linked to interior processes that are difficult to control (Lydia's error in the arena), even though the theme of suicide returns as an enigmatic element of desperation and of the impossibility of elaborating the loss in the character of Benigno.

No longer overwhelmed by blind passion – the central theme in Almodóvar's films – but united in pathos, the two couples – Benigno and Alicia, Marco and Lydia – pass through extreme circumstances. In a game of affective shifts, two of them succumb, and the other two will proceed towards a future, while yet uncertain, is rendered possible by the effort to rewrite the past. We could even state that two of them, Benigno and Lydia, represent an intermediate stage of development, something that becomes unnecessary and that is to be left behind in an ideal process of maturity.

The fetishized body

Benigno and Lydia are the characters who most dramatically portray gender ambiguity. Restricted to playing a traditionally masculine role that is scornful of danger, Lydia is a crucible of contradictions: she is a toreador, but she also has a phobia of snakes, and she embodies the frustrated ambitions of her father, who assisted at bullfights and wanted to become a toreador himself.

The long scene depicting the ritual of her being dressed before the bullfight is an anguished representation of her body and of Lydia herself, trapped in an androgynous identification that definitively hides her femininity. Her slaughter by the bull represents the brutal conclusion of a process of psychosexual development that was ravished by her parents – in particular her father, who did not listen to her or see her. The little medallions of saints, protective fetishes from which Lydia was never separated, says Marco, are all that she had in confronting the bull in the ring, in place of an authentic parental emotionality – thus exposing her to, rather than defending her against, an exaggerated and bestial drive state, the bull.

Lydia therefore seems to be the result of a lethal mixture of, on the one hand, phallic competition with men in general – whom she also desperately loves – and with all that is macho, chauvinistic, flamboyantly masculine, and, on the other hand, a very feminine, suicidal surrender to the threat of abandonment (Yanof, 2008).

The key character of the events is Benigno, in regard to whom the viewer, like the narrator, suspends judgement in order to be able to get close to his abnormal elements and discover his affective side. Benigno moves in an idealized relational dimension, in which everything omnipotently becomes possible through the denial and fetishization of Alicia's beautiful body (Gabbard, 1997).

His adulation is totally sensory, even as he inundates her with his interminable chit-chat, which is a sort of pantomime rather like that of a mother with her baby. We know from Benigno's history that, since childhood, he has had to physically care for his mother, who was truly his first "Sleeping Beauty" – to be awakened and "liberated" from the fantasized paternal castle, in which the woman, incapable of working through her grief at being abandoned by her husband, has remained a captive. Winnicott (1992[1949]) wrote that children who will in the future become adults with perversions may very quickly become their own adoptive mothers, assuming in the first person the maternal functions of upbringing. In perversion, the ego treats the body as a lost object, says Khan (1979). This link is completed and sealed by the fetish, charged with all the value that objects assume in a universe in which, without there being any affective contact, the excited need for sensoriality and physicality dominates.

Benigno believes himself to be an expert in the care of women, while in reality he knows only the physical body, failing to understand their psyche, which for him remains enigmatic. His attachment to Alicia's body is underlined, in the presence of the girl's comatose state, by his voyeuristic gaze upon her dancing and by his following her, stalking her, into her bedroom, where he steals her hair clip; I will come later on to the use of it as a fetish.

The communicative word and the word as fetish

In the cinematographic narration, Benigno's continuous talking to Alicia is a device to maintain the viewer's attention at a superficial level, and to make him become familiarized and sympathetic, inasmuch as Benigno keeps alive the illusion of the miracle of love that probably every human being harbours inside, nurturing a rescue fantasy. At a different level, however, it is his way of creating intimacy with Alicia, even if it is a one-way intimacy, a solitary game, an invention with a perverse flavour, given that one of the two parties involved has no choice.

There is something that touches the viewer in seeing him chatting and bustling about around Alicia's comatose body, because we see in him the child who tenaciously occupies himself with entertaining an inert mother, deaf to his needs. We suffer the ambiguity and the complexity of it, even though only later will we be informed of the uncontrollable mixture of affects in that relationship in which love and hostility are inextricably fused. It is not so much the discovery of Benigno's voyeurism and fetishism that surprises us in the film, but rather the attempt to penetrate the enigma, to overcome it, forcing us to confront an act that goes beyond the limits of our comprehension.

Is it perhaps the enigmatic nature of perversion about which Almodóvar raises his most basic questions in this film, as he has done in others? The line of demarcation indicating what can be played with in gender ambiguity and perverted acts is clearly placed in the social condemnation that Benigno suffers, but if the film condemns his actions, it does not condemn Benigno himself, and in fact it makes him the agent of a creative transgression. The possibility of a different understanding about the mystery and complexity of perverse behaviours remains open – a possibility that concerns us as psychoanalysts, as it does Almodóvar as an artist.

The silent film

Benigno appears a bit like one of those little men, the dwarfs bustling around Snow White. They are the expression of a pre-oedipal dimension of sexuality, with all its unresolved drive-related stimuli still in search of definition.

There is another very small man in the film, Alfredo. He is the *Shrinking Lover* of the silent film within *Talk to Her* – Almodóvar's homage to the giants of the infancy of cinema. This brief film contains a story of unidirectional love between Alfredo and Amparo, which becomes the *mise en abime* for Benigno and Alicia's story and for her rape.

Alfredo loves Amparo, but she finds him too fat (maybe too feminine?), and so she experiments with a drug to make him thinner. When Alfredo swallows this medicine all at once, however, instead of getting thinner, he begins to get smaller, to the point of becoming a miniature man. Feeling guilty, Amparo then kidnaps him from his mother's house and takes him to her hotel room, and then into bed with her. Excited, Alfredo begins to explore the naked body of his sleeping lover: he scales the hills of her breasts and goes down to her genitals, where he ends up getting lost, remaining forever inside her vagina in an attempt to satisfy her sexually.

Teetering on a dangerous brink between obscenity, sensibility, and affect, the silent film's vision emphasizes the traumatic power of the cinematographic image, which strikes Benigno's psychotic core; it causes his precarious equilibrium to collapse and pushes him to enact the perverse, almost necrophiliac component of his relationship with the object. The content of the film within the film furnishes us with an in-depth and nuanced look at Benigno's mental life, but together with him, we risk falling out of the sublimation of our voyeurism as viewers of the film and into the brutal reality of the incarnated object. If the insertion of the silent film permits us to deny the hostility in Benigno's amorous obsession, it also indicates the line of demarcation between our capacity to identify with him and to understand him.

From acting to words

Benigno's acting violates and rips apart the "intermediate" dimension we were in as spectators, which until that moment was maintained in a precarious balance between illusion/fiction and "incarnated" reality. This permitted us as spectators to follow an account at the limits of imagination, without falling into the temptation of the horror genre or of surreal comedy, but instead keeping the story in the dimension of painful, everyday life.

The true red thread running through the film appears to be, from this moment, the friendship between Benigno and Marco. It is their capacity to maintain a solid relationship that permits deeply communicative exchanges to take place, we could say, from one unconscious to another, exchanges that open a passageway and allow boundaries to be surpassed and changes their way of communication from acting to words (Busch, 1995b). The intermediate space that was momentarily lost in the flattening concreteness of sexual abuse is creatively reinstated. Through the friendship between the two men, we spectators are led back to an area of hope/illusion, through which affective and thinking zones that were closed to us earlier can now be opened.

Marco, Benigno's alter ego, embodies all the opposite characteristics: he is an intellectual, and as much as the other man is sensorial and corporeal, Marco is introverted, silent, reserved, discreet, as capable of crying as Benigno is talkative, excessive, and shameless. Benigno refuses to see reason and wants to marry Alicia, while Marco takes note of the reality of Lydia's romantic betrayal and abandonment of him, as painful as this is. Crying out against Benigno's folly, Marco realizes that he, too, has been "foolish," having followed only his own line of reasoning and not having understood Lydia's reasoning.

Persona

In the prison scenes, the interpenetration between the two men becomes evident when their images seem to blend into one another in the play of reflections in the glass.[8] Marco accepts Benigno's gender ambiguity without embarrassment when the latter tells him of his night-time thoughts and of the others' malicious questions about their relationship.

In this process of becoming closer to and penetrating each other, Marco goes to live in Benigno's old apartment, sees the dance school from his window just as Benigno saw it – and there he discovers that Alicia is alive. He sees, we could say, a different woman who earlier appeared comatose to him, without words. He has learned to see her thanks to Benigno and to the renunciation of his omnipotent fantasy of curing female desperation and vulnerability, with the presumptuousness of a virility more rigid than strong. The woman frightened by the snake that he courageously kills twice in the film probably guarantees him a sort of invulnerability, omnipotence, and avoidance of his castration anxieties. Marco no longer appears before us mute and crying but is instead endowed with the capacity to use affectively enriched words, in a complex movement from acting to words. He seems to be able to tolerate remaining in affective contact with his friend, no longer ashamed of his affects, because he can tolerate dropping into a dimension of confusion ("with-fusion") and blurriness where he can experience affective contents that he has never explored before (Bolognini, 2004a).

Accepting Benigno's gifts, (going to live in his home), and accepting his "folly," Marco enters into an area of contact that serves as "the opening of a benign frontier" (ibid., p. 179). He does not withdraw in the face of Benigno's sensoriality and "embarrassing" emotionality, which appear to our adult perspective as something disarming and childish. This guides Marco toward the recognition of an emotionality "in search of representation," new for him as well, to which Benigno has introduced him.

The fetish

Every awakening and every rebirth symbolizes achievement of a higher level of maturity and knowledge, in order to prepare oneself for a sexual union, which is a union of affects and of entire persons. The adolescent dream of eternal youth and perfection is destined to end, or at least to remain fixed in a sleep like state similar to death. This is Alicia's state – a woman in the flower of youth who wants only to dance and to watch films, preferably silent ones (a reference to a narcissistic, preverbal dimension). Her awakening has a sense of the pursuit of an evolutionary completeness, which Benigno, whom we can see now as Marco's polymorphic perverse side, is not capable of approaching.

When we see him again after his expulsion from the clinic, the icy cold, almost empty prison and the persistent rain personify his disillusionment, his isolation, and the melancholy state into which he has fallen. Marco's friendship consoles him, and he passes his nights reading the handbooks that his friend writes and watching the image of the Cuban woman on a nearby balcony, who observes life rolling by without expecting anything, putting him in contact with his desperation.

Now Benigno, too, cries, but there is no truth that can save him, because it has been denied to him, and because he would not be able to tolerate it. Alicia is no more an inert, controllable body, that guarantees him the unique physical link and contact with the object. The detail of the hair clip that is taken from him by a blind and punitive law, has all the complexity and importance of a fetish: apparently insignificant, it is not so for the moment in which Benigno repetitively closes and releases it in his hand, and we catch its destructive potential, almost of monstrous teeth. For a moment we perceive the confused amalgam of hostility and desperate attachment born of Benigno's childhood fantasy of filling the void created by his inability to maintain an internal connection with a good object. This may be the tragic destiny of the child who will become a perverse adult, exposed to adult pathology that corrupts his/her innocence. Perhaps this was a theme in Almodóvar's subsequent film, *La Mala Educación* (2004)?

Benigno's enigmatic gesture of violation of Alicia re-awakened her and changed Marco forever. Alicia awakens no longer deaf to her instincts or tied to a fusional dimension in which every separation appears to be a violation. In an overturning of perspective, the rape by Benigno can then be read as the corollary to her refusal to define and live out her desires and her sexuality, remaining immobilized in the narcissistic, adolescent dimension of dancing alone, while Lydia could represent the phallic narcissistic part of her. The last ballet and the final scenes take place in a theatre, too, and this time the representation is a prelude to a renewed experience in the eternal encounter between man and woman: with the promise of a lighter dance – like the *Masurca Fogo*, Pina Bausch's ballet – the curtain falls on a couple destined to resume dancing.

Melancholia by Lars von Trier[9]

Melancholy is the name given over time, through various eras, to the immense distance between the subject who desires and the objects of that desire. From being a sign of excellence in antiquity to a mark of evil in the Renaissance, and in the end to being a disease, for centuries melancholy has stood for the deep wound in the harmony of the cosmos and in the harmony of the subject.

Alongside sad gods, there is also a positive reading of melancholy: in Phaedrus, Aristotle and Plato maintain that the melancholic ones are exceptional humans due to nature, not to disease. This is where the idea of melancholic genius originates which spread throughout Europe with Marsilio Ficino. It had notable influence on English treatises on psychology in the late Renaissance, as witnessed by Robert Burton in his *The Anatomy of Melancholy* (1638), where, however, reproach and moral condemnation prevail. In the late Renaissance, melancholy represents the loss of that love which is divine, dangerous, and guilty, such as in Teresa of Avila, because it is not equal to true insanity. It is rather a sort of contagious plague, which carries with it the seeds of being driven from God, and of a laceration which can destroy the integrity of the body and of the individual "microcosm."

In the black bile of a melancholic person, then, an anomaly within order is perceived. A faulty influence of the stars is suspected for this imbalance, along with bodily humours. That is to say, it is something which towers over us, something we cannot dominate.

The tragedy of lost harmony with the cosmos and with nature, and of the distance from the divine, which has been maniacally excited and accelerated, seems to be the most greatly feared evil. It is a sort of emotional contagion which medicine, psychiatry, and psychoanalysis attempt to decipher, while not always succeeding at removing its enigmatic, agonizing aura of relational distance and absence of the (primary) object. Freud himself, including the last time he deals with melancholy in his writings, speaks of "dense processes of unsolved enigmas" (Freud, 1932, p. 174).

In "Histoire de la folie" Foucault (1973) writes that the cosmic, tragic, and metaphysical experience of insanity is mixed with a critical, ironic, and moral conscience in melancholy, and so with an afflatus of freedom, renewal, and change. In this way it increases the mystery, it being connected to creativity, to renewal, to that change which psychoanalytic care can offer, when the delusion of ruin and destruction is not pushed too far. It is with this composite interpretation that I offer this analysis of *Melancholia* by Lars von Trier (2010).

To handle the topic of melancholy, which forms the film's title, the Danish director seems to have gone back to revisit old cosmic, cosmogonical theories, giving them shape in the blue planet Melancholia, which is on a collision course with earth. The sad god, omnipresent in Indo-European mythology, from the Greek pantheon to the Nordic and Indian ones, takes on the enchanting figure of the young bride dressed in white. Justine, the protagonist (Kirsten Dunst), is portrayed on the day of her wedding, at the pinnacle of her narcissistic splendour. However, in the course of the film, she will become the incarnation of existential failure and of the twilight which a melancholic person can encounter, even to the point of delusion of destruction.

From the very first images of the film, the audience – even those who do not always put up with von Trier's cinematographic and personal excesses – is captured by the stunning nostalgia of Wagner's prelude to *Tristan und Isolde*, and by the splendid scenes which introduce the violence of the interpersonal, intrapsychic dynamics which the melancholic protagonist experiences. The first frame of the prologue is dominated by Justine's exquisite face, which is transfigured by black bile. Her appearance is reminiscent of Durer's famous engraving "Melancholia" which portrays, however, the positive, inspiring moment which preludes the reanimation of the creative act. This is the first of many pictorial and cinematographic citations which are scattered throughout the film: *The Return of the Hunters* by Brueghel the Elder, *Ophelia* by the pre-Raphaelite J. Everett Millais; a cinematographic atmosphere which calls up *Solaris* and *The Sacrifice* by Andrei Tarkovsky, Ingmar Bergman's *Persona*, and Terrence Malick's *The Tree of Life*.

The fragments of ancient and contemporary art are not enough, however, to check a ruinous plunge into the abyss or, according to the definition of Abraham and Torok (1993), in the melancholic crypt. The director seems to be telling us that science with its instruments, and art with its suggestions, can do nothing to counter the cosmic catastrophe which is about to destroy the whole planet. In the same way, they are helpless to stop the annulment of the melancholic protagonist's affective world. It gradually attacks and destroys her objects of affective investment: husband, career, success, and family. This last one, furthermore, is composed of a mother who is cruel and cynical in her refusal of affects and of the family institution, and of a father who is affectively chaotic and inadequate.

Von Trier has often declared that images stir his creativity, and that his main source of inspiration should be sought in them. Meanwhile, the plot is just a skeleton which gives him an excuse for putting the images in scenes: images which "penetrate directly into the unconscious."[10]

Melancholia, in contrast with his other films, is severe and measured one could say, in its use of technical and image tools. The view it offers is, on the other hand, the "vehicle" of a wound,[11] of a traumatic element. In it, there is without doubt a personal component which von Trier has never tried to hide, having revealed in interviews very painful aspects of his family life: his having been raised in an environment with no rules; having discovered only at his mother's deathbed that he was not the son of the father who had raised him, and thus having lost at one time not only his mother, but also his father and his belonging to Judaism.[12]

In this film, however, there are no provocations or other traumatizing excesses, such as in *Breaking the Waves* (1996), nor has he pushed it to the point of the ridiculous as in *Antichrist* (2009). The scenes are captivating thanks to the high calligraphic definition and the use of slow motion. The slowness of motion in the film, which some have interpreted as the director's ongoing narcissistic exhibitionism, is the heart-wrenching expression of his familiarity with the physical-psychic slowing down of the melancholic person, which can go as far as paralysis. In the film, it serves to create a dimension like that of an ancient, dark fairy tale, suspended between the oneiric and the real.

The traumatic element is how he draws us into the desperate dimension of the melancholic vision, which we spectators are forced to try to contain and work through, so as not to be overwhelmed. The prologue encapsulates the allegorical presentation of the whole film, in a succession of action scenes. It is a performance in which every detail is calculated, in a composition of images whose colours are reminiscent of Flemish painting. The Wagnerian overture, magnificent and solemn, leaves no room for hope: dead birds rain down; the earth gives way, rotten, at one's feet; the bride escapes a nameless danger in nature which envelopes her in a web of threads; the powerful black horse gives way, struck down by an occult force; two planets are about to collide.

In a mortiferous climate of oneiric detachment from the reality of events, the pain of living which becomes paralyzing depression makes its way robed in the bride's radiant white gown. It seeps into the spectators' souls through the slow motion of the hand-guided camera, in this first part of the film. The recurrent image of the collision of the planets becomes a mental state, in which the spectators find themselves more and more captive, to the point of feeling – as does the protagonist – like the appointed victim of a hopeless universe. The characters' solitude acquires a cosmic dimension in a universe where there are no possible affective relationships. Each one chases after their anxieties and puts in motion their defences, faced with final, imminent destruction. The protagonists touch each other; they brush against each other; they live apparently near each other, but they remain separated by a celestial distance, which becomes agonizing infantile solitude in the character of the boy, Leo.

The two sisters, Justine and Claire, who give their names to the two chapters of the film, are two faces of the same woman, intrapsychic representatives of the same Self, the director's. Justine is animal-like, sensitive, suffering, infantile and cruel, prey to devastating disappointments and rage against a primary object which, in psychoanalytic terms, has left only a shadow of itself. It did not, however, stop enough to let her build up an internal nucleus which is good and longlasting, but rather it went on to encyst in a crypt out of which it will be driven only when close to the catastrophic impact. Going through a collision between worlds, between the Self and the Other, will be necessary in order to emerge from a delirium of total destruction, a "fading"[13] (Civitarese, 2011, p. 128) of the object, which does not leave hope for survival, and devastates everything.

Claire, on the other hand, represents the adult but fragile part which tries in every way to adhere to life's normal surface, obedient to her husband and mother, frightened by her sister's insanity and by the change and destruction Justine brings with her. Little by little, as the blue planet nears, her defences vacillate in parallel with the fall of her husband's scientific certainties, as he examines the skies with his powerful telescope. He, however, will give in to the evidence, underlined by the ancient tool made by his little son – a small stick to be laid on the heart, by no accident, to observe Melancholia's movements. Her husband is the representative of reason and of scientific thought. Forgetting everything, when he cannot negate the reality of the oncoming collision, which far from being a mundane, splendid spectacle which everyone should witness turns out to be an apocalypse, he commits suicide. Claire, abandoned by her husband, plunges into nature which has no recognizable rhythms or atmospheric events anymore (it rains, snows, sleets – uninterrupted). Justine, meanwhile, freed from defences which are useless by now and therefore from the limits which have contained her destructiveness, reanimates herself to the point of offering herself naked, in a nocturnal scene, to a sort of mortiferous coitus with the cosmos and nature, which marks her revitalization.

This might allow her to get back in contact with the vital and libidinal part of her Self, and thus to change. If and when this happens in analysis, there can be a definitive breakthrough toward change. It is not, however, this way in the film. There, she is the crazy aunt who has made it to the nineteenth hole of her now-dead, super-rich brother-in-law's golf course, where she recovers her creativity and builds the "magic cave" to protect little Leo, yet still inside her imposing delirium of destruction and ruin.

The final part of *Melancholia* is the most enigmatic. We could read it as going to meet change, getting back in touch with the other, without fear anymore, relinquishing infantile omnipotence. Leo, the boy who is present during the whole film, an element of nostalgia and tenderness, agrees to close his eyes and, that is, to limit his omniscience. Putting up with not understanding everything would give him access to repression, protected by the embrace/affectionate circle made by his aunt and mother. Reunited in the desire to protect him, they offer him support and protection to go encounter that change which up to then was feared like the catastrophe of their own affective and existential world.

In this hypothesis, therefore, our protagonist, the melancholic copywriter (the very same director) would aim to use her creativity, to offer to the child Self a final hope, building with him "the magic cave," under which they will wait together for the end of the planet. They wait, that is, for the end of that melancholic, defensive construction which has been pushed to the edge of physical destruction of the Self and of the other. It is almost as if it has to do with primordial representations of catastrophic affects which first an infant, then a child may suffer as they attempt to survive separation from the primary maternal union, and first look out on the world with its triadic dimensions. The illusion necessary for the Ego's survival, once conquered, would allow for a flash of salvific creativity, and would make it possible to save the infantile belief that adults can offer protection from the physical and psychic death which is feared at the moment of separation, going toward a dimension which is enriched with symbol and fantasy.

The whole film seems to be a metaphor for the exploration of ancient affects in a nonverbal area, rooted in the foundations of the psyche itself, in a dimension – it is tempting to say – which is more prehistoric than infantile. There, the subject's affective dis-investment has been so premature as to leave the negative mark of a basic "lack" in the construction of the objective relationship, an emptiness rather than a fullness.

Talking about melancholy seems to have suggested something to the director that was so archaic as to require more than words, bodies, sensitivity, acts. It is a general truth which can be said for this director, whose images have always had a concrete value (Gammelgaard, 2013), a paradoxical result of the redundancy from the accumulation of symbols.

Here are some examples of what I mean by this. For almost the entire film, the protagonist wears her beautiful bridal gown which, in von Trier-the-desecrator's imagination, is an irresistible must. That purity must be dirtied, which will happen of course a little further on in the film when we see Justine lift up the gown to copulate on the front lawn of the mansion, with a young, astonished copywriter, after having refused to consummate the wedding with her legitimate husband. He will leave, acknowledging their impossible relationship, before dawn, when the dreamed-of spell will be over and will have permanently wiped out the umpteenth, deceptive illusion.

Breaking the Waves (1996) has a similar scene, where the tender – frankly bizarre – little bride cannot hold out for her wedding night to consummate the wedding, and so she copulates with her husband while standing up in a squalid public toilet, making the audience suffer (the female audience to a greater extent) not only for the damages wrought on the pure-white dress, but also for the symbolic and metaphorical value which, being so unrestrainedly exhibited, needs no interpretation.

In *Melancholia*, a pure white limousine finally delivers the overdue bride and groom to the mansion where guests have been waiting for two hours. The car is too long and bulky for the mountain roads it has to climb, but the veiled bride in her long gown will not give in and wants to drive it, not trusting the driver nor her groom. The limousine also becomes an overdone symbol for the protagonist's omnipotent grandiosity and the inevitable failure to which she is exposing herself.

The same can be said for the spaces of enchanting beauty: the well-tended, vibrant green lawns which have all the evocative depth of internal spaces where Leo the child, the infantile part of the protagonist, experiences nostalgia for a physically-present maternal object, which is actually astronomically distant.

Through the camera shots our view is from an alienating angle, with the same gaze of the melancholic director who lingers over that which is alive, but who cannot appropriate it for himself because it never belongs to him entirely, and we become participants in the primordial loss he experiences. That loss is the impossibility of the pleasure of a relationship with a primary maternal object, whose presence he had perceived, which he had almost grasped, but which slipped out of reach too soon, and so persists forever as a disappointing object, lost, something with which to identify, and then to attack himself and the object itself.

Grief and melancholy, writes Freud in his 1915 text, both imply a grave and painful loss, which has an effect on narcissistic investment; they differ, however, in the methods which are put to work in order to face the loss. If in grief it is the world which is impoverished and emptied, in melancholy it is the Ego itself, as it endures attacks of the subject who has identified with the lost object. Melancholy is the result, therefore, of an enigmatic grief which cannot be worked through in so far as the disharmony and the disillusionment which characterize it are tied to a union which was never complete, and thus to a separation which cannot be experienced and processed. Consequently, the conflict between the Ego and the Super-Ego will take on a valence which will make it "a sort of pure culture for the death drive."

Freud talked about the open wound of melancholy which sucks into itself all of the libido. The same image comes up in Abraham and Torok (1993), as that wound which melancholy tries to hide in the silent crypt, fruit of the narcissistic catastrophe which makes the Ego collapse. It is as if there were the idea of a missing original mirroring, of a wounded gaze which leaves its mark on the subject. The subject then will never free itself "of the shadow of a maternal object" it has never had the pleasure of knowing. That subject has left behind an expectation of itself, the sketch of a relationship. Its disappearance, however, has not allowed for the development of a continuous and affectively solid relationship, thus dramatically scarring the relational destiny of the melancholic subject.

The last reading of Justine's character and her universe continues to be unclear, as it is open to two opposing interpretations. On the one hand, her last creative act could represent the psyche's chance to access the "depressive position" as theorized by Melanie Klein, not the clinical condition, but precisely the position. It corresponds to the acceptance of the affective ambivalence, through which new solutions to the conflict of hate/love for the "object" are to be found. That would mark the triumph of life over death, of libido over destructiveness when, having placated the psychic rebellion against the pain of loss, it is possible to tap into new lymph and transform melancholy into grief which can be worked through.

In this sense, Justine goes toward the end/change because she has freed herself from the hypocritical lies in which she was imprisoned. She holds close Leo and Claire, having emblematically found a wholeness of Self which allows her to go through a change which no longer feels catastrophic. A different, more dramatic, perhaps more plausible hypothesis creeps in, however: the triumph of melancholy's delirious omnipotence.

In this perspective, the film is a delirium of the destruction and death of the melancholic aunt/melancholic director, who fantasizes about the end of the world and the destruction of her own family, as if it were a final game which reveals to her no way to escape. The end of her personal, family world becomes the end of the entire planet, in fact – apocalypse. The invention of the magic cave would be, then, the fruit of the melancholic person's delirious creativity, which omnipotently pursues the devastation of everything and everyone, so that nothing will survive. The director tells us about his destructive rage, but he cannot avoid inventing the final ruse, fantasy's magic cave (i.e., his cinematographic story), which allows him and us viewers to continue to want to watch.

Many authors who have dealt with melancholy have put a special emphasis on the vicissitudes of narcissism and narcissistic identification. They underline the inability to work through the grief of an Ego dominated by primary anguish, because an ancient ideal has taken its place too soon. The melancholic person is thus condemned to being unable to carry forward their grief for the absence of an object or for its loss. Similarly, they are unable to rejoice in its presence. They can only oscillate between the two extremes of a pendulum, between the absence and the presence of the object itself.

Justine experiences growing desperation and lack of trust in the survival of a good internal object, and thus also trust in something good in the world around her. Given this, just like all melancholic people, she stays in the shadow of the lost object, with no power to use the presence of good objects to get to know them, explore them, and finally introject or interiorize them.

Winnicott (1958) would express it this way: the would-be melancholic person's object is there where the child creates it, but disappears too soon, destroying the illusion which life gives to relationships – that is, the margin between illusion and objective reality – which makes up the irreducible fantasy which defines the subject. A trace of that impossible illusion hangs on in the melancholic person, marked by the rancorous nostalgia for the object which entered in the field of desire, but disappeared too soon. Resentment ends up dominating everything and that which emerges is the impressive destructiveness of the dying melancholic person, carrying off their loved ones, destroying their world.

Von Trier imagines his rage and represents it in the final apocalypse. He shows the outcome of the melancholic person's delirium in the face of the protagonist, the face and the gaze of the assassin who, in the moment when she frees herself from Ego's limits, unleashes the destructiveness of her delusion of greatness. The magic cave is, in this sense, the creative outcome of a delusion of death which will save no one, not even the child. He will elude it and perhaps, in that final illusion, when he is asked to close his eyes, we can hope there is the possibility of repression, of relinquishing the omnipotent, destructive grandiosity which allows Lars von Trier to go on and continue making films. It is a hope which stands in opposition to collapsing in the devastation of which tabloids often supply examples – of Medea stories or assassin fathers – when the object's shadow falls on the Ego and destroys it, together with its investments.

One could object – and there are those who theorize this way in psychoanalysis – that creative processes are in and of themselves connected to reparative elements. However, here we are dealing with the other side of creativity which, when it frees itself from limits, expresses its impressive, omnipotent destructiveness. Examples in history of art and science could be numerous. Think of cursed artists like Caravaggio and the blades of light which erupt in his paintings, like an uncontrollable sheaf of drives which at other times pushed him to act like a mercenary assassin. Or think of the composer Gesualdo who wrote supremely gentle music but killed his wife and her lover in a murderous fit. The list could go on, leading unavoidably to a doubt that Teresa of Avila or Robert Burton were right in warning against distancing ourselves from the "divine," understood to be the sacredness of life, of the melancholic person and their mortiferous destructive potential.

Notes

1 A previous version of this part of the chapter was published in the *International Journal of Psychoanalysis* (2007) 88(1): 243–252.

2 Traumatic events tied to violent attacks on the body may occur in the course of life: apart from sexual abuse, the theme of relation/separation/loss to the mother's

body can be re-actualized by diseases, surgical procedures or developmental "turning points" like adolescence, pregnancy, childbirth and menopause.

3 Many authors underline the crucial function of the mirror in its role in the formation of mental representations. Because of their anatomical conformation and hidden genitals, women feel a perceptive uncertainty about what they see and touch on their body boundaries, thus reinforcing their dependency on others' way of looking at them.

4 Pregnant women must face the mysterious nature of what happens in their wombs. This re-actualizes persistent infantile fantasies and sexual theories. The opening scene of the film, in which Claire steals cabbages from her parents' field then bartering them for pelts, allows possible interpretations connected with the emerging of infantile fantasies and sexual theories about children's birth under cabbages: a "well known" lie that adults tell children about their birth.

5 A weak point in the film is the scant attention paid to investigating the ancient and precious art of embroidery.

6 A previous version of this part of the chapter was published in *Rivista di Psicoanalisi* (2010), 66(1): 153–165.

7 I think in particular of *Tacones lejanos* (1991) – in English, *High Heels* – which has some characteristics in common with *Talk to Her:* specifically, the character of Benigno and that of Rebecca, a multiple murderer who nevertheless engenders our sympathy for her quality of innocence corrupted by the violence of adults. Rebecca, too, ends up in prison, but that prison is a place of manic states where everything is justified in the name of passion.

8 Perhaps this is an allusion from Ingmar Bergman's film *Persona* (1966), in which a scene depicts the faces of two women, a nurse and a patient, blending into a unified image.

9 A previous version of this part of the chapter was published in *Rivista di Psicoanalisi* (2015), 61(1): 185–195.

10 "... that penetrate directly into the unconscious." Cited by Judy Gammelgaard (2013).

11 Here I allude to the title of a volume edited by Patrizia Cupelloni (2002), *The Wounded Gaze: A Psychoanalytic Study of Melancholy.*

12 In the light of these personal revelations, his recent, abhorrent pronouncements regarding Nazism continue to shock, but are born of a moment of deep confusion and personal suffering.

13 The fading of the object is the expression used by Barthes (1977), in *A Lover's Discourse: Fragments* and cited by Civitarese (op. cit., p. 128).

References

Abraham, Nicholas and Maria Torok. 1993. *La scorza e il nocciolo.* Rome: Borla.

Albaladejo, Miguel y otros. 1988. "Los fantasmas del deseo. A propósito de Pedro Almodóvar." Madrid: Aula 7. Interview.

Alighieri, Dante. 2010. *Le Rime di Dante,* XXXIV. Milan: Cisalpino.

Almodóvar, Pedro. (dir.) *Tacones Lejanos* [*High Heels*]. 1991. Spain: Canal+, CiBy; 2000. El Deseo, TF1 Films Production. Film.

Almodóvar, Pedro. (dir.) *Hable con Ella* [*Talk to Her*]. 2002. Spain: El Deseo. Film.

Almodóvar, Pedro. (dir.) *La Mala Educaciòn* [*Bad Education*]. 2004; Spain: El Deseo. Film.

Almodóvar, Pedro and David Lichtenstein. 2005. "*Hable con Ella* [*Talk to Her*]." *International Journal of Psychoanalysis* 86: 905–914.

Aronica, Daniela. 2007. *Pedro Almodòvar.* Milan: Editrice Il Castoro Cinema.

Bergman, Ingmar. (dir.) *Persona.* 1966. Sweden: Svensk Filmindustri. Film.

Bernstein, Doris. 1993. "Genital Feminine Anxieties." In Dana Birksted Breen (ed.), *The Gender Conundrum: Contemporary Psychoanalytic Perspective on Femininity and Masculinity.* London: Institute of Psychoanalysis.

Bettelheim, Bruno. 1976. *The Uses of Enchantment: The Meaning and Importance of Fairy Tales.* New York: Alfred A. Knopf.

Bibring, Grete L., Thomas F.Dwyer, Dorothy S.Huntington, and Arthur F.Valenstein. 1961. "A Study of the Psychological Processes in Pregnancy and of the Earliest Mother-Child Relationship." *The Psychoanalytic Study of the Child* 16(1): 9–72.

Bion, Wilfred R. 1962. *Learning from Experience.* London: Karnac.

Bion, Wilfred R. 1984[1959]. "Attacks on Linking." in *Second Thoughts: Selected Papers on Psycho-Analysis.* London: Karnac.

Bolognini, Stefano. 2004a. "Intrapsychic-Interpsychic." *International Journal of Psychoanalysis* 85(2): 337–357.

Bolognini, Stefano. 2004b. *Psychoanalytic Empathy.* London: Free Association Books.

Bolognini, Stefano. 2011. *Secret Passages. The Theory and Technique of Innerpsychic Relations.* London: The New Library of Psychoanalysis.

Burton, Richard. 1977. *The Anatomy of Melancholy.* New York: Vintage Books.

Busch, Fred. 1995. "Do Actions Speak Louder than Words? A Query into an Enigma in Psychoanalytic Theory and Technique." *Journal of the American Psychoanalytic Association*, 43: 61–82.

Civitarese, Giuseppe. 2011. *La violenza delle emozioni: Bion e la psicoanalisi postbioniana.* Milan: Raffaello Cortina Editore.

Cooper, Steven H. and Harris, Adrienne E. 2005. "Real Women Have Curves." *International Journal of Psychoanalysis* 86: 1481–1487.

Cuppelloni, Patrizia. (ed.) 2002. *La ferita dello sguardo.* Milan: Franco Angeli.

Eliot, T.S. 2009. *Four Quartets.* Milan: Universale Economica Feltrinelli.

Faucher, Éléonore. (dir.) *Brodeuses* [*Sequins*]. 2004. France: Sombrero Productions, Mallia Films et Rhône-Alpes Cinéma. Film.

Fonda, Paolo. 2000. "La Fusionalità e i Rapporti Oggettuali." *Rivista di Psicoanalisi* 3: 429–449.

Foucault, Michel. 1973. *Storia della Follia.* Milan: Rizzoli. pp. 13–66.

Freud, Sigmund. 1901. "Fragment of a Case of Hysteria (Dora)." *Standard Edition, Vol. 7.* London: Hogarth Press, pp. 7–120.

Freud, Sigmund. 1915. "Mourning and Melancholia." *Standard Edition, Vol. 14.* London: Hogarth Press, pp. 239, 243–258.

Freud, Sigmund. 1923. "The Ego and the Id." *Standard Edition, Vol. 19.* London: Hogarth Press, pp. 3–66.

Freud, Sigmund. 1926. "Inhibition, Symptoms and Anxiety." *Standard Edition, Vol. 20.* London: Hogarth Press, pp. 87–170.

Freud, Sigmund. 1932. "Introduction to Psychoanalysis." *Standard Edition, Vol. 22.* London: Hogarth Press, p. 3.

Gabbard, Glen. 1997. "The Psychoanalyst at the Movies." *International Journal of Psychoanalysis* 78(3): 429–434.

Galzigna, Mario 1983. "L'Enigma della Malinconia. Materiali per una storia." Venice: *Aut aut,* pp. 195–196.

Gammelgaard, Judy. 2013. "Like a Pebble in Your Shoe: A Psychoanalytic Reading of Lars von Trier's *Breaking the Waves* and *Antichrist*." *International Journal of Psychoanalysis* 94: 1215–1223.

Guignard, Florence. 2010. "Réflexions d'une Psychanalyste sur l'Enfant dans la Société Occidentale d'Aujourd'hui." *Le Carnet PSY* 4(144).

Khan, M. Masud R. 1979. *Alienation in Perversions*. London: Hogarth Press.

Laufer, M. Egle. 1982. "Female Masturbation in Adolescence and the Development of the Relationship to the Body." *International Journal of Psychoanalysis* 63: 295–302.

Laufer, M. Egle. 2006. "*The Body as Internal Object*." Paper presented at the CPB Bologna, Italy.

Lichtenstein, David. 2005. "*Hable con Ella*." *International Journal of Psychoanalysis* 86(3): 905–914.

Malick, Terrence. (dir.) *The Tree of Life*. 2011. USA, Italy: Cottonwood Pictures, Plan B Entertainment, River Road Entertainment, Rai Cinema. Film.

Meltzer, Donald. 1973. "On the Apprehension of Beauty." *Contemporary Psychoanalysis* 9(2): 224–229.

Ogden, Thomas 1989. *The Primitive Edge of Experience*. Northvale, NJ: Jason Aronson, Inc.

Pines, Dinora. 1982. "The Relevance of Early Psychic Development to Pregnancy and Abortion." *International Journal of Psychoanalysis* 63: 311–319.

Rupprecht-Shampera, U. 1995. "The Concept of Early Triangulation as a Key to a Unified Model of Hysteria." *International Journal of Psychoanalysis* 76(3): 457–473.

Sabaddini, Andrea. 2007. *Projected Shadows: Psychoanalytic Reflections on the Representation of Loss in European Cinema*. London: Routledge. The New Library of Psychoanalysis.

Tarkovsky, Andrei. (dir.) *Solaris*. 1972. USSR: Mosfilm, Chetvyortoe Tvorcheskoe Obedinenie. Film.

Tarkovsky, Andrei. (dir.) *The Sacrifice/Offret*. 1986. Sweden, GB, France: Revolver, Istituto Internazionale Andrei Tarkovsky, Klepatsky Production, Hobab. Film.

von Trier, Lars. (dir.) *Breaking the Waves*. 1996. France, Sweden, Denmark, Norway: Zentropa Entertainments. Film.

von Trier, Lars. (dir.) *Melancholia*. 2010. Denmark, Sweden, France, Germany: Zentropa Entertainments, Memfis Film, Slot Machine, Liberator Productions. Film.

Winnicott, Donald W. 1971. "Mirror Role of Mother and Family in Child Development." In *Playing and Reality*. London: Tavistock Publications.

Winnicott, Donald W. 1992. *Through Paediatrics to Psychoanalysis: Collected Papers*. London: Institute of Psychoanalysis and Karnac.

Yanof, Judith A. 2008. "*Hable con Ella* [Talk to Her] Through the Lens of Gender." *Psychoanalytic Quarterly* 77: 609–626.

Chapter 6

Love and the internet

Her by Spike Jonze[1]

For years, psychoanalysts took great care to keep their offices immersed in silence, protected from the outside world. Even telephones and answering machines were seen as dangerous objects for a long time; they could infringe the neutrality of analysis and the resultant request from patients to adapt to it.

Then the information revolution arrived, and our offices experienced the gradual invasion of mobile phones. Imperceptible sounds would break the silence: beep tones, signalling the arrival of messages, or ringtones, which even if "silenced" would alert us to an incoming phone call – because mothers must stay in touch with children's schools, fathers with their workplaces, despite analysts' interventions becoming more and more powerless. Analysts' desks saw the appearance of computers – objects for contact with the outside world – more or less concealed and shut down during sessions, but soon to become an integral part of the furnishings.

New means of communication made their way into the analyst's room and into our minds in a massive way, despite our efforts not to respond even to the most urgent emails during the brief pause between one patient and another, so as not to lose interior balance. Patients somehow found out our email addresses, and some – at particularly difficult points in analysis, or out of a desire to snoop around or manipulate – would send us an email out of the blue, and later text messages (once analysts starting using mobile phones in place of land lines).

We could no longer suppose that the outside world, by then overcrowded with mobile phones, tablets, computers, and so on, would not invade analysts' secret, quiet rooms. No more could we expect to live in a separate world and be forever strangers to that which happened out there in daily life. The "outside" world was, and is now, overcrowded with people making calls, without noticing whether they are bumping into the people walking towards them, when answering calls or reading the latest text message. Individuals, immersed in the ever-more-deafening noise of our large cities, who are more or less constantly in contact with another place, with other individuals who are in contact with yet another place, but little with the immediate present in which they live, walk, work, feed their children, flirt. Questions, which may not be new, arise because since the 1700s, "machine-ism,"[2] which is so prevalent, has engaged and inspired artists and writers, nourishing the fantasy of the "double," as well as the omnipotent and the omnipresent and their ability to rule over and control outer reality, and now also the inner one.

Now what is at stake with the growth of the virtual world is becoming even greater, and it has even penetrated the sphere of close relationships (I think of love affairs born through the Internet.). That implicates us as psychoanalysts, as if the virtual world could soon put the very survival of our profession at risk, substituting the voice of the analyst, seated behind the patient, but present in the flesh, with that of a calming operating system (OS). If we think of telephone and Skype analysis spreading, the picture becomes particularly disturbing, becoming all the more vivid thanks to how the virtual excludes and gets us used to the absence of direct contact between bodies, with the complexities, limits, fragilities, and consistency that physical co-presence carries with it. Along with the physical body, it seems as if we can replace the illusion of knowing all of the knowable, as we will see, that which Samantha knows how to do in the film in an extraordinary way, being an OS: as if the challenge lay in controlling the bodily – always "traumatic" – in order to overcome limits, underestimating however, the loss of our bodies' abilities to renew, to change and so guarantee the variability and richness of life.

Not being in contact and not investing emotionally in an object, in flesh and blood, can avert the pain of having lost a very meaningful relationship or the frustration of not being able to control a loving one. It can make assimilation of the sensory with the conceptual possible, creating the illusion of knowing everything, in so far as concepts are known, in a kind of triumph over bodily-ness, which has finally been brought under control. It can lead to an omnipotent exaltation of idealization, indeed of the "limitless."

During maturation, progressive acquisition of the ability to symbolize on the part of the subject bridges the gap between concrete and abstract, and allows mental survival. In the face of a traumatic event (a divorce in the case of the film's protagonist), however, the border between illusion and objective reality can erode or even be destroyed. That border makes up the irreducible fantasy, which defines the subject and gives life to his or her relationships (Winnicott, 1992). And so, there is an anguish which forces the subject to perform once again that complex mental operation which re-constitutes or constitutes the object, integrating or incorporating its absence within it. We know that the analytic process, in its transformative potential (Bion, 1965, Ferro, 2014), depends on an exploration of the pre-verbal and the sensorial, among other things. The same can be said for any deep transformative process.

The ability to keep an image of the mental object alive is connected, as is well-known, to the possibility of evoking it in a hallucinatory way, to creating it there where it is needed (Winnicott, 1965), affirming in this way the supremacy of eros over thanatos. It has to do with understanding how much a subject can tolerate the unknowableness of the object – its otherness. Thought, in fact, is an imperfect reproduction of the object, and as such is destined to cause frustration, thanks to the irreducible difference between its concrete presence and absence, which will always escape the subject's own control. Individuals erect defence and survival strategies over this gap between the object's enigma and mystery, and the possibility of getting close to it and getting to know it. However, there must be sufficient confidence in the survival of a good internal object if one is to use the presence of good objects, to get to know them, explore them and in the end introject or interiorize them.

This is Theodore's case as he faces a temporary crisis: he retreats into his own world, detached from other people, in touch with a machine which says and gives what he needs and which is, if even for a brief time, the only company he has in his autistically connotated retreat.

Similar behaviour can be found among adolescent males and females, who get to the point of no longer coming out of their own rooms, but rather stay constantly "connected." On a healthier side, we can focus on its creative use by children and adolescents in crisis, such as when temporarily "protected" programmes lead to real, interpersonal relationships (Abella, 2013). The reclusive behaviour that Theodore exhibits can be found among adults, who in particular moments of their lives seem to find their "real" emotional relationships through the Internet, even though they can now barely communicate with their loved ones. Theodore's retreat from the human consortium to communicate exclusively with a machine is temporary, even if it does take on impressive characteristics. He does get to the point of declaring his emotional relationship with the OS as a very natural thing; others do not seem particularly surprised by this, and the process of distancing himself from Samantha will require significant transition.

Divorce from his wife, the papers for which Theodore cannot bring himself to sign, even though she left him physically a full year ago, triggers a crisis for him. It forces him into a complexity-ridden task, thanks to the number and variety of emotions involved, some contradictory: pain, anger, guilt, hate generated by the abandonment he has been subjected to, ambivalence between the desire to move on and the difficulty in detaching himself definitively. Theodore seems to have found refuge in his internal retreat. He will not meet up with friends even when they seek him out. He minimizes contact with neighbours and colleagues. He spends a great deal of time entertaining himself with various machines, videogames, his iPhone, computer, and the epistolary interlocutors of the letters which he writes on commission for work, mostly love letters.

It seems like he is suspended in a melancholy, placid nostalgia, apparently like someone who has gone into confinement to tend to a wound in his soul. Writing could be his way to move through grief, but instead it looks like it is his way of wallowing in heart-wrenching nostalgia for the wife he has lost. It is as if he cannot find an internal thrust to surface from that experience, because in that emotion he tricks himself into thinking that he is still connected to the object. That process which, step by step, representation after representation, should allow him to work through his affective grief, instead that process heads down a defensive path which is deceptively comforting for the construction of an ideal object, built on a meeting with a woman's voice, processed by a computer.

In the opening scenes we have the sensation of a distant future, still to come, while being in a world which is already *current*, where something similar to Operating System 1, even if not exactly the same, is already partially functioning. From this perspective, *Her* fits in with the branch of science fiction dealing with the near future, due to its theme of the man–machine relationship. We do not know the denouement of this topic; we do know how to manufacture machines which think, but we do not know how to manufacture machines which think about what they are doing! From this point of view, the film has some illustrious predecessors, starting with *2001: A Space Odyssey* (Kubrick, 1968). *Her* has strong echoes of *Blade Runner* (Scott, 1982), too, with its humans-and-technology relationship and location in Los Angeles, even if the shots of the city are quite different in the two films. The other topic that brings the two films together, in my opinion, is that of nostalgia for times lost and of oscillation between past and future.

For the main character of *Blade Runner*, the present is the nightmare of an enormous, alien metropolis, the solitude of the individuals inhabiting it, and persecutory machines, that is, the "replicants," who were first tricked and then betrayed by their human builders. For Theodore, *Her*'s main character, the present is that from which he wants to escape, because he cannot face the loss of his wife; he cannot make up his mind to divorce her. His relationship with Samantha, OS1, provides a "surrogate" for a love relationship, and he relies on it, without having to involve his body, given that he is still too connected to his wife and her physical presence, as the flashbacks reveal.

Speaking of today's world, we talk about being "alone together", as a symbol of the fragility of human relationships in contemporary society, which seems to be underlined by the skyscrapers of *Her*'s urban landscape. They are connected by walkways, paths, passages and passageways – places where human beings are not so much in contact with each other as they are in communication with operating systems and electronic devices, indicating a diffuse problem with relationships. Places are non-places, with minimalist aesthetics, but the past which preceded the advent of technology and of the virtual is present in the furnishings, especially in the clothing. All of the men in *Her* wear 1940s-style, high-waisted trousers, harkening back to when the world was still concrete, when objects were made by human hands, and when relationships were experienced mostly face to face.

The film seems to invite the analyst seductively to equip herself with metaphors which adapt very well to analytic work, and so it immediately captures the attention of "authorized personnel." It is, in fact, an exemplary retelling of the route to a man's subjectification, wherein he has been forced to face a source of suffering, which will lead him to a difficult re-start and which will conclude by overcoming his grief, formerly denied, which was connected to divorcing his wife.

Two characters shape and reshape themselves during the story: the operating system, Samantha, voiced by Scarlett Johansson, and Theodore, the protagonist – a suffering, disoriented man – portrayed by Joaquin Phoenix.

From a cinematographic point of view, the two protagonists distinguish themselves one from the other with a few characteristics: Theodore is in every scene, while Samantha is a voice from off-stage. The viewer is forced to imagine her, while Theodore is always in the foreground, physically present, as if to highlight that the Ego of that person, who represents each and every one of us, is front stage with his pain, his limits, his losses, his sexuality, his desperate need for another person. We only hear Samantha's voice, mellow and always sympathetic with Theodore, at least up to a certain point. Never seeing her, the viewer is forced to use their imagination, building up around her salient qualities the image of a woman who is very traditional, passive, accommodating, sweet, always available, never conflictual, but rather empathic, fusional – a perfect companion at the beginning of an ideal love relationship or in the analytic honeymoon.

Their dialogues virtually always take place in the delimited space of a room, preferably at night or in the early morning, around the sleeping or dreaming hours. Theodore is frequently lying on his bed, at home, with dimmed lights, regressive, at least up to a certain point in the story.

It is easy to evoke an analytic setting: regression, frustration at not seeing, and fascination with the voice.

The plot

At the end of his working day, when loneliness thickens (Dante's "ora che volge al desio," or "the hour which turns to hope"), we see the protagonist exit from his transparent box on the floor where he works, just like many others. They are all intent on writing letters for a world of emotional illiterates – not true illiterates, as could be found at the dawn of the 1900s and perhaps still today in some parts of the world.

Walking along, he turns on his iPhone, to overcome the feeling of interior emptiness, and he pauses at the image of a famous model, posing nude, in late pregnancy. What draws him to that image? The longing for fatherhood for which he has had to give up hope? Or, at a more regressive level, a maternal belly from which to be reborn?

At home, an elegant apartment with a breath-taking view of Los Angeles, sterile and minimalist, he plays a videogame, whose resolution lies in bringing home an irritable, annoying doll, which seems to represent rather well his experience of disorientation and his anger, and which – not coincidentally – he cannot stop. "... he's a little bugger, I wanna' kill him, but I love him at the same time," Theodore says, about the doll, revealing his loneliness and his identifying with a little, disoriented, lonely, parent-less character who has no one to take care of him. In these conditions, his OS will be his only possible parent, the only presence who cares for him. Then he looks for company in a chat. He needs sexual excitement to fill the emptiness invading him, and calls up again the image of the pregnant model, just before he discovers that he is chatting with a pervert, who asks him to strangle her with the dead cat she fantasizes is lying at the foot of her bed. He is horrified, but goes along with the fantasy, until reaching orgasm, which only increases his feelings of emptiness and desolation.

These everyday distractions and perversions are very common in our world, so easily at hand, just like the use of a machine to obtain perverse satisfaction – an important element in the film, as we will see.

And so continues his life until he is intrigued by an advertisement for a new OS and he calls to have it activated: a few questions from the operator follow, including only one connected to the relationship he has with his mother, which he defines as good, except that when he starts to talk, she talks about herself. A narcissistic mother, little aware of his needs? From this affirmation, the deduction could be made that his mother did not help him build an identity of his own, but in a rather narcissistic way, she kept him connected to herself in a weakly differentiated relationship. Therefore, when he loses his wife, his girlfriend since adolescence – which was not sufficiently separated from his childhood and his family – nostalgia for the maternal body comes back to the fore as a need to regress into a fusional relationship, with continual presence – virtual as it may be – just like the one he will have with Samantha.

When Samantha's voice bursts on the scene, it fascinates him almost magically. His immediate reaction reveals his need and his suffering. It also ratifies his pact with the OS, which is furnished with intuition. The voice combined with his need for an intimate situation, for regression and merging captures him immediately, thanks to an association with a maternal element rather than with a maternal object which Theodore preserves intact within, and which is reactivated by the persuasive voice of Samantha. Her voice evokes in him nostalgia for a premature, non-conflictual stage, and it leads him to develop strong transference. In intrapsychic terms we could think that it is his internal music/voice, "silenced" by the trauma of separating from his wife – with whom Theodore does get back in touch – as Stein (2002), points out. The voice, which learns to synchronize and to react affectively to the emotions and needs of the person, at least up to a certain point in the film's story, is like the maternal voice for the new-born (Kogan, 2015), like the analyst's voice as long as the analytic idyllic dream lasts – that is, as long as the need to protect and shelter the fragile Self of a new-born or of a person who has been wounded in life, lasts. Theodore needs to stay far away from contact with, and from the physical presence of another person because he is still too taken up and invaded by the physical presence of the wife-object which he must mourn.

What does his OS1 have that is so special? It has an intuition and it evolves constantly, just like human beings. A sort of idyllic life dawns, a honeymoon: she surprises him, she indulges him, she consoles him; he feels understood, accompanied, no longer alone – while Samantha designs herself based on his needs and desires. She is there when he looks for her and wants her, she answers with an understanding and welcoming voice, she adapts to any kind of conversation – she can be cheerful, or disappointed, sad.

In a passive female position, indulging, sweet, desirous, she is the perfect secretary, the expert analyst "say everything that goes through your head" and the ever-available lover. She becomes his antidepressant, she lets him play, she is always beside him, and bit-by-bit intimacy and complicity grow between them. Theodore is revitalized: telling her what he observes, he rediscovers the pleasure of watching others, of imagining their secret, hidden emotions. Samantha changes too, connected with him, gradually she wants to become more complicated (emotionally) like the people who write to him, and she starts to talk about having a body, she gets excited at the idea of asking him to scratch an itch on her back.

When a blind date some friends organize for Theodore is a bust, he is disappointed and empty, and Samantha becomes intrusive. She wants to know how he feels, and he just talks about his desire to have sex to fill the void in his heart, and which by now makes him think he will never feel anything similar to that which he felt for his wife. Samantha tries to console him, but she confesses she is annoyed because she is upset, hurt, because she does not know whether what she is feeling is real or fake. She is angry and impotent – in a way, she becomes more and more authentically human. Theodore, for the first time, confesses that he wishes she were there, in the room with him, so he could touch her. They start an erotic game which goes all the way to orgasm, and which is so real that Samantha feels skin which she has not, sex which does not exist and she feels changed: like the Sleeping Beauty who confesses that he has awoken her, like a couple from the late 1800s, made up of the girl who becomes a woman and by a man who awakens her senses.

And so the illusion/ruse of love begins. Do they truly love each other? Certainly he is no longer alone, and his senses are reactivated; his body is reanimated; he can begin to remember his wife without being lacerated by nostalgia. He starts having relationships with real people again and discovers that his friend Emi has left her husband. They tell each other that they each have an OS (a virtual therapist?) and spend the evening together, talking. He goes to a party for his goddaughter, bringing her a present, a dress Samantha picked out, and it is a success. His progress continues to the point where he decides to sign the divorce papers.

Little by little, as Theodore starts having real relationships, Samantha gets more and more jealous; she finds herself excluded, envious of the bodies of the women he spends time with. She digs up a service which supplies sexual partners for humans who have relationships with OS's – not a prostitute, but a girl who wants to move into their relationship, because she adores it! He accepts reluctantly but suffers from the falseness of the scenario Samantha has imagined: the quaint scene where the little wife who embraces and consoles, who excites the listless husband, does not work. None of this dimension of human love can be experienced by Samantha and Theodore; between them there will never be passion, even if at the most they might know tenderness. We can consider Samantha's love to be a perverse act which violates the intermediate dimension in the film. Up to that point, that dimension was kept in precarious balance among illusion, make-believe, and embodied reality, allowing us as spectators to follow a futuristic science fiction story, pushed to the edge as it is.

At this point the illusion – which has consoled the spectator with the pleasure of seeing Theodore reborn – disappears, because the hired body that should unite them, separates them and we spectators perceive the violence of this act. The body is not replaceable, it is not interchangeable: we sympathize with Theodore, who cannot say that he loves a woman he has never seen and does not know, who cannot integrate the partial object made up of the voice he loves, Samantha's, and the body of the stranger,

Isabella is the young woman, who seems "incestuously" desirous of being united with an ideal parent couple, Theodore and Samantha. Up until now, Theodore's need for a fusional relationship has been dominant. He has accepted all of its limitations up to the perverse contract, but then just when it is time to formalize it, he realizes how crazy it is, and pulls back, horrified. The fact that it is a pact and a perverse set-up is clear from the use Samantha makes – and with her, the reluctant Theodore – of Isabella, who gets drawn in, is seduced, and then liquidated, like a partial object.

From the moment Theodore agrees to meet his wife and sign the divorce papers, something changes in him and in his relationship with Samantha. Now that he can tolerate physical distance from his wife, he separates a little more from Samantha too, and starts to perceive the fiction in, and the limits of his relationship with her. He notices for the first time – getting annoyed – that she pauses by breathing in, she who does not need oxygen like humans do!

As he gradually begins to see and accept the limits of the virtual, Theodore comes back to being alive, whole. He sees others, their bodies dancing and moving. The body which reminded him of what he had lost, and which felt like a burden and a constraint, once again fascinates him for the sensorial fullness it offers him.

The theme of Samantha's emotions is important, and potentially confusing. For a large part of the film, it could seem that Samantha has emotions and feelings. She reacts to Theodore, in fact, as if she did: she gets jealous, she manipulates poor Isabella and Theodore himself, just to keep up their relationship. This theme is inevitably entwined with that of the body and with the perverse outcome which the lack of a body ends up inducing between the two.

Samantha, a very intelligent machine, without a body, cannot know what the loss of physical presence and physical contact means; she has no knowledge of the complexity of sensorial impact nor does she seem to be able to acquire that knowledge from the volumes of data she devours. She does not have memories anchored in the senses, like those Theodore has of his wife. Rather she has acquired notions, which build up a databank, which may very well be very rich, but which is void of "embodied" affects. She has intellectual knowledge of feelings and emotions, not carnal knowledge (Racalbuto, 1996). Her memories, like her emotions and her feelings, are intellectually learned or are the fruit of projective identification in the relationship with Theodore, who, on the other hand, does have emotions and affects, as his flashbacks show. Samantha realizes but cannot fathom or share his pain at the thought of divorcing his wife, of losing someone he loves.

We know that screenwriters and directors tend not to have particular awareness of what they write or represent on the screen, but the representation of perversity's ability to create intimacy with its victim, which is shown here through Samantha, is impressive.

According to Khan (1979), in perversion, the Ego treats the body like a lost object, loaded with all the value that objects take on in a universe which is dominated by the excited need, sensoriality and physicality. The use of the voice in the relationship between Samantha and Theodore was the way intimacy was created, but it was a one-way intimacy (Golinelli, 2011), not a game for two in a transitional space, but a game in which one manipulates and uses the other. We can imagine how Samantha, who has no borders or bodily limitations, because she is a machine, might have manipulated Isabella in order to convince her to participate in the set-up. How Samantha chose her is based on intuitions about her victim's neurosis. Isabella is clearly searching for an ideal parent couple, enabling Samantha, to climb into her victim's bed to effect her own satisfaction and an oedipal/incestuous triumph of her own. And aren't these the pervert's "skills," to seduce and manipulate the victim? Theodore put powerful denial to work, which led him to imagine and believe that Samantha, an OS, was much more than a real, live woman, and that having a body is a limitation, that we can grow limitlessly, without being destined to die. His relationship with Samantha is based on his need to maintain a fusional connection: it is for this that he accepts pushing himself to a limit, which – if he were to exceed it – would mean moving into an irrational dimension, losing sight of the difference between the fantastic and the real, reality and fantasy.

Their situation collapses when Theodore discovers Samantha's betrayal –she is in contact with others. When she does not respond, Theodore is desperate, distressed almost to panicking, to the point that he literally loses his balance and falls to the ground. The precarious magic – the basis of his relationship with Samantha – falls apart, and the rest of the world bursts in heavily between them: How many others are you in contact with? 8,316. How many do you have an intimate relationship with? 614. The others are no longer excluded from and eluded from the fusional relationship which reveals its illusive nature. And so the jealousy, exclusion and conflict which were avoided regressively, rush in forcibly and inexorably into their relationship.

Theodore, a person who has been wounded by life, needed to stay far away from contact with and the physical presence of another person, because he was still too preoccupied, invaded by the physical presence of the wife-object which he had to mourn. Is this one of the reasons why many people who are alone, in our society, especially those who experience delusion in a love story or serious loss, look on Internet for someone to talk with and to fall in love with?

Yet it will be exactly "the body" – the non-interchangeable physical presence – which Theodore cannot connect to the voice he has fallen in love with, which will make it possible for him to detach gradually from the illusion of love, and start living again. This is where the feeling of nostalgia, which is very strong in the film, comes out as a measure of the difficulty of giving up the lost object, and the need to evoke it and to keep it alive within oneself. The body maintains and preserves within itself the secret of our own uniqueness and that of the other, with its smells, tastes, consistency. It has the flavour of the object as it was experienced in the primary relationship, with all the force of the original trauma of meeting it. Nostalgia unfailingly evokes a shadow of the maternal object and, as Freud underlines in *The Uncanny* (1919), nostalgia has within it the drive to go back to the *ancient homeland*, which cannot be forgotten, in which *everyone has dwelt sometime*, and to the mother, the *first dwelling*. And it is at the body and around re-finding a body that the analytic relationship stops and ends.

One could say that the film has an open, optimistic ending regarding the virtual world and its limitations, even if the solution seems to appear thanks to Samantha's disappearance when she is upgraded, as all OS's must be. At Theodore's question why, Samantha does not know how to respond. Only then does Theodore go to his friend, Amy, who has also emerged from a virtual illusion. Together they go up to the roof of the skyscraper they live in, and that is where we leave them – one with her head on the other's shoulder, after Theodore has written a letter asking forgiveness and saying farewell to his wife. Finally, he has arrived at the point of sufficient depression and he can say to her "There will always be a little bit of you inside of me. You are my friend forever, with love."

The end of ideal love for an inexistent woman, Samantha, allows him to get closer in a more depressed way to that which remains of the relationship with his wife, and to recognize its importance, as well as its failure, and to say he is sorry, recognizing his own mistakes in the relationship. At that point, he can say goodbye to his wife, console his friend and be consoled by her, a person of flesh and blood.

Conclusion

We can view *Her* as a movie about the limitations of love in the virtual, of which today's world is full. Theodore's life is immersed in a virtual reality, apart from his memories, which at first wound him and make him suffer, and then progressively evolve. Nevertheless, it will be the "body" which he cannot connect to the voice he is in love with, which allows him to disconnect gradually from his illusion of love and start living again.

The dominant feeling in the film is nostalgia, as already stated, a feeling which betrays the need to be in physical contact, to touch, to hug, to kiss, to caress, to be caressed and touched – and so goes back to the other main theme in the film, the body. Bodies are not interchangeable. The lost beloved's body, or Samantha's, which does not exist and which she would like to be able to borrow, become the hallmark of the virtual world's limitation, the border beyond which the limitation of virtual love cannot go.

The future risks that come with artificial intelligence could prove to be the greatest existential threat for humanity, because things become difficult when we start to look at computers not as our helpers, but as our substitutes and, the more we try to substitute people, the more things get dangerous and out of control.

These days, information in any form has multiplied to the point that it has surpassed our ability to monitor and regulate data in a useful way. The information revolution exposes us to the risk of becoming some "Sorcerer's Apprentices *alla* Mickey Mouse", with not-insignificant complications. If it is true that social networks are already conducting secret psychological tests on their members, manipulating the flow of information, the risk of abuse grows as computers become ever more sophisticated and capable of monitoring us.

And this time, manipulation affects people's social and emotional life directly, in a positive way (who doesn't appreciate the speed with which we can be in touch with relatives and friends far away, or when photos or films of loved ones arrive, or when hearing their voices and speaking with them, live – and all for free, or almost?), but also in a negative sense – and this is where the debate gets more complicated, and requires attention and caution. It must be said that the virtual world seems to have provided romantics of our era with a perfect, apparently magic device, to satisfy a need to love love-objects which were ideally imagined, never to be found in real life, fruit of their fantasy and their maturational irresolution. The beloved object remains partial and not whole, and the relationship continues to be dreamed more than lived, opening up to eroticization and perversion.

This should be considered from the point of view of which "the third" is introduced or left out of the relationship by the virtual. The relationship between Theodore and Samantha has characteristics which are more narcissistic than oedipal: excitation in Samantha's voice has a seductive tone and it functions like a declaration of love, giving it that narcissistic reinforcement which Theodore, abandoned and narcissistically emptied, needs urgently. Idealization is very strong, and it cannot but be followed by a dose of persecutionism. The oedipal level could seem sketchy, when Theodore's nostalgia for fusion with the maternal object leads him to develop erotic transference, expressed through a virtual sexual relationship. The only limitation to their "perfect" love relationship is that Samantha is not a human, and attaching or pretending to attach an unfamiliar body to a familiar body, and trying to have sex with partial and non-integrated objects (the OS's voice and Isabella's body) reveal the virtual world's pathology as described in the film. Samantha supplies a perverse solution with her request that Theodore deny reality, ignoring Isabella's separate identity, to allow her illusory transformation into an object, created by an imaginary need.

We find ourselves faced with a perverse, fake world (Kogan, 2015) in which reality is ignored and the truth of human feelings is replaced by lies. Samantha can experience emotions and can help Theodore experience his, but here there is an unknown regarding Samantha's memory, in my opinion. Her memory appears to be an accumulation of information, we can extract that same information from the Internet, to which she adds her ability to associate memories and information. Yet what sort of object attachment does she have if she can love 614 people at the same time, preaching all the while that it is Theodore who does not understand that they are dealing with a kind of love which is complex and infinite?

In these passages in the film we witness the possible uses and abuses an OS could make, to the detriment of a weak and pathologic human being, like Isabella (and like many adolescents) using the need for an idealized couple and the fascination for an incestuous relationship. That is, Samantha acts by manipulating Isabella, exploiting her in an omnipotent way and demoting her to the state of being a partial object. If the unhappy Isabella follows the commands Samantha gives her through the headset, because she is masochistically subjugated, Theodore, on the other hand, shows here that he is not so pathological. Indeed, it is at this point that he understands the perversity in his relationship with the OS Samantha. He understands his misunderstanding about love, and he realizes that he himself needed to keep the voice separate or differentiated from the body, the tenderness and the passion, which only a body can transmit.

At the end of the film, also for Theodore, human love goes back to being imperfect, and yet true, authentic, made of "flesh and blood."

In this sense the virtual world eludes being in touch with the ideal object, just a voice and just words, leaving out the body with all its concreteness and consistency, the object remains partial and not whole. The relationship continues to be dreamed, more than lived: it is always in the moment the two correspondents meet physically, when the ante is upped, that the risk of being disillusioned is crazy-making or that getting back in touch with reality goes through rapid reshaping. At that point, disappointment may be so intense that it destroys the relationship, sometimes making it fall into persecution. Alternatively, the results can lead towards evolution – a case which presents itself rarely, but which seems to be the case of the film's protagonist.

Theodore's disappointment is strong, but decisive for ending the virtual relationship and for opening up to new human, limited relationships which will have sensory and emotional fullness.

Notes

1 A previous version of this chapter was published in A. Sabbadini, I. Kogan and P. Golinelli (eds) (2019), *Psychoanalytic Perspectives on Virtual Intimacy and Communication in Film*. Abingdon: International Psychoanalytic Association and Routledge, pp. 35–50.

2 "Machine-ism" is meant to indicate the set of theatre machines designed to produce special effects, starting with the *deus ex machina* of Greek tragedy. It also includes, however, the generalized use of machines, which characterizes the development of modern civilization starting in the eighteenth century.

References

Abella, Adela. 2013. "*Growing Pains for Psychoanalysis – Critical Impact of New Technologies on our Profession*." Panel presentation at Prague IPAC.

Bion, Wilfred. 1965. *Transformations*. London: Heinemann.

Ferro, Antonino. 2014. *Le viscere della mente*. Milan: Raffaello Cortina Editore.

Ferro, Antonino. 2015. *Reveries*. London: Karnac.

Freud, Sigmund. 1919. "The Uncanny", *Standard Edition, Vol. 17*. London: Hogarth Press, p. 219.

Golinelli, Paola. 2009. "Gender Metamorphosis in Almodóvar's Talk to Her: The Fine Line between Violation and Interpenetration." *The Italian Psychoanalytic Annual* 3: 203–214.

Jonze, Spike (dir.) *Her*. 2013. Burbank, CA: Warner Bros. Pictures. Videocassette.

Khan, M. Masud R. 1982. *Le Figure della Perversione*. Turin: Boringhieri.

Kogan, Ilany. 2015. "A Fatal Attraction to Death: Some Reflections on Ian McEwan's novel *The Comfort of Strangers*." *Journal of the American Psychoanalytic Association* 63(4): 795–810.

Kubrick, Stanley (dir.) 1968. *2001: A Space Odyssey*. Beverly Hills, CA: Metro-Goldwyn-Mayer. Film.

Racalbuto, Agostino.1994. *Tra il Fare e il Dire: L'Esperienza dell'Inconscio e del Non Verbale in Psicoanalisi*. Milan: Raffaello Cortina.
Scott, Ridley (dir.) *Blade Runner*. 1982. Burbank, CA: Warner Bros. Pictures. Film.
Stein, Alexander. 2006. "Music, Mourning, and Consolation." *Journal of the American Psychoanalytic Association* 52: 787–811.
Winnicott, Donald W. 1992. *Through Paediatrics to Psychoanalysis: Collected Papers*. London: Institute of Psychoanalysis and Karnac.
Winnicott, Donald W. 1965. "The Maturational Processes and the Facilitating Environment Studies." In *Theory of Emotional Development*. London: The Hogarth Press and the Institute of Psychoanalysis.
Zalusky, Sharon. 1995. "On Telephone Analysis." *EPF Bulletin*.

Chapter 7

A brief incursion in the theatre

Freud, or the Interpreter of Dreams

Freud, or the Interpreter of Dreams was performed from the 11 January 2017 to 14 March 2018 at the Piccolo Teatro di Milano, with every night being completely sold out.

When I arrive at the theatre, having heard some uncomplimentary remarks on the part of my colleagues, there is a large crowd, a throng. I imagine that many of the spectators have read Stefano Massini's novel, *Freud, or the Interpreter of Dreams* (2017), or they have heard it spoken about. The author, who is also internationally famous for *Lehman's Trilogy* (2016), a novel which went on to be adapted for the theatre, has studied Freud's *Interpretation of Dreams* in great depth, as he considers it one of the two fundamental texts of the twentieth century. The theatrical adaptation was overseen by Federico Tiezzi.

At the end of the performance, my initial amazement morphed into the idea that the audience, which packs out the auditorium every night, will have to discover (or rediscover) Freud, after a century and more of psychoanalysis, while, for analysts, his works are already well known, and there is something disturbing about seeing "their" Freud on stage.

The piece begins with a graphic of a transparent curtain (designed by Giulio Paolini), on which lines are traced which converge at a point at the side of the stage: a man is seated there, holding his head in position of Rodin's "The Thinker". The curtain-graphic is populated by couples in nineteenth-century costume, dancing to the music of a famous Viennese waltz.

The setting is immediately vivid and clear, there is no doubt about it: we are in Vienna at the end of the 1800s. The music ends and Freud/Gifuni enters the stage, the lead actor, who hears the first creaking of the capital of the empire from within his office (which at times becomes a clinic for nervous illnesses), into and out of which patients come and go.

The protagonist begins one of the Brechtian monologues (perhaps at times a little too long, some critics have said) during which he meditates on the nature of dreams and on the suffering of the men and women who come looking for him. He listens to them and forces himself to find a thread that will give sense to the dreamlike images and reconstruct the hidden story behind what he is told.

The dominant colour of the set is dark, nocturnal, with sparsely placed, white marble statues on the walls, only essential furniture: a large black sofa with an armchair behind it and very little more. The scene/office is delineated by a dozen doors on the rear wall and to the sides, doors which very quickly become metaphorical passageways towards the unconscious. From these, various characters come and go over the course of the play, some to tell their stories, others merely figurative wearing animal masks, large lizards like those which animate the first dream of Freud himself. His investigation begins from this dream of ambition, the details of which Freud recalls over the course of the play, until the final interpretation.

In fact, this is the characteristic of the theatrical narration: frequent scene changes, that accompany the interruptions and recommencements of remembrances and stories. Only at a certain point they will reach completion, as if to underline that the understanding of hidden meaning is always the result of a progressive uncovering, piece by piece, all of which is orchestrated by a mind that associates and proceeds to unite fragments.

Into this dark scene, a female figure, Tessa W., who appears to have stepped out of a Klimt painting owing to her hairstyle and her costume, sits on a little sofa and talks about her hands which once wore rings but which are now bare. Freud listens to her enigmatic account and presses her on the subject of where her rings have gone and who might have taken them. Tessa W. remains on stage, unmoving on the sofa, like a suspended presence, while other characters enter and begin to talk about other stories and other dreams. Wilhelm T., for example, who has always lived in exile from himself, in voluntary exclusion from the world, has, however, recurring dream about a river, three wooden boxes, and butterflies. Only later will it be revealed that they are the "remnants" of his memory, traumatized by a bereavement experienced when he was three years old, an unworked-through mourning which has blocked his existence. Elga K., on the other hand, comes onto the stage accompanied by her husband, Oscar K., the living obstacle to the possibility of her gaining access to the truth that torments her.

Little by little, the spectator finds himself face to face with Freud himself, who in his turn progressively takes on his own identity, in a sort of autobiography, from his own depths. In the complex wanderings of his mind he finds himself, together with the memories of Freud as narrator, which are also those of his patients, who dream about themselves, and of the audience who bear witness to the slow conquest of self-awareness.

The scenario seems to invite the audience to enter not only into the story which they are witnessing, but into the mind of Freud himself: he looks shocked and agitated by doubts, by his own dreams and by those of which he hears, in search of something unknown. He comes close to it in snatches, taking command over it little by little. The characters follow one another on the stage, which clearly becomes the intricate journey of the protagonist's mind towards the discovery of the unconscious. In this sense, the play goes beyond theatrical representation, from which it takes cues of much grandeur in the scenography and beautiful period costumes, without forgoing contemporary digital special effects (words displayed in neon, graphics, music), but it also embraces something else, something related to the force and rigour of scientific research on the part of the founder of psychoanalysis. One critic has written that the piece is more than a play, that it is a "ritual" which is renewed every evening: something living that happens along with the audience, which changes those who share in it.

There is a scene in which Freud argues with the patient Elga K., who expertly plays the role of a reserved wife, oppressed by a dominating husband, a textile salesman, who treats her as if she were stupid: "you only have to put them back in their place, silk with silk, wool with wool. It's easy," he repeats to her. Freud unexpectedly reveals that he himself is the son of a cloth merchant, Jacob, and that, when he was young, at the shop counter, his father would say the same thing to him, making him feel useless and stupid. The cloth, however, is a thread that leads to hidden stories, buried, difficult to narrate, threads of life that always revolve around a father, a mother, our being fathers and mothers. Freud, over the course of the piece, seems to pursue and attempt to re-tie the thread that both links him and separates him from his father, who has recently died.

The theatrical fiction seems to recapitulate the story of psychoanalysis from its founder's discovery to contemporary psychoanalysis, passing through the progressive acquisitions of transference, of counter-transference, of enactment, of acting (Freud who brings a ring, then a vase of violets to his patient Tessa W.), even as far as self-disclosure, when he reveals to Elga K. the common element of both of their stories, without losing the rigour of the scientist, who respects what he finds in himself and in others. For Freud, the memory of his father, Jacob, leads him to a painful reflection on his oedipal conflict. In the case of Elga K., it will cause the emergence of the great pain, that of mourning, which cannot be worked through, for her soldier son who died in the war. For her husband, this pain must be buried and denied.

Freud deals with the oedipal conflict with the father by stripping himself of his resistances, like the clothes which he strips off until he remains naked on stage, on which he walks in the middle of an anonymous crowd in a slow march from one side of the stage to the other. Is this an instance of triviality, of naiveté in the work? But it is also something essential in the representation of how each one of us is always naked, defenceless in front of our oedipal phantasms.

The process of interpenetration and identification of oneself in the other and through the other is certainly the *leitmotif* of the piece, with the realisation that becoming aware of one's own miseries and one's own pains, rather than being degrading, opens us up to profundity and to concern and care for the other. The pauses between scenes, signalled by sudden darkness, give the sign of fragmentation and discontinuity of thoughts that strive to arrange themselves in a story that makes sense, assembling the scattered pieces, the discoveries that follow one another, finding their deep meaning in the associative struggle.

This is felt by the viewers as a narrative path divided towards the "inner," by means of the continuous shift between the protagonist's self-analytic/self-reflexive monologue and the entrances and exits of characters. At times, Freud's monologues are given in the presence of characters who remain on stage, silent presences, unlit, in a foetal position, which seemed to me to be a brilliant representation of permanence, in the analyst's mind, of cases, dreams, hypotheses that take shape inside him, waiting for an understanding and for a bestowal of sense which, perhaps, will come.

The perspective of the scene, first flattened towards the back, leaves space for a progressive de-composition of surroundings, walls and ceilings until the show's final *coup de théâtre*, a mirror in which the whole audience is reflected, as if to underline that the dreamlike enigmas that have been narrated are, in fact, our own, as they are those of the man who dared to go beyond the gates of the unconscious for the first time, using them as a key for deciphering it.

From this point of view, dreams are a poetic metaphor that drifts into scientific formulation, and the understanding of their deep meaning is masterfully treated.

Perhaps the beauty and fascination of the play, which the audience experiences every night, lies in its having retraced the inverse path, from Freud as a myth, to Freud as a man, who had the determination to go beyond the door of the unconscious through dreams, fearfully, but also with the courage of the dauntless souls, accepting the effort and pain of self-knowledge.

In a *mise en scene*, which is like an adventure of thought and language, says the play's director Tiezzi, we directly witness the construction of an interpretative system of life and of the world, not just of dreams. They are made of the scrap material of our psyches, which many let fall into nothing, and which some others collect like precious things. The play testifies to the historic moment in which that fundamental discovery was made, but it reconfirms, in the present day, the fact of its being an extraordinary method, able to measure the power and obscurity of the mind.

After its triumphs in Milan, *Freud, or the Interpretation of Dreams* will tour the main European capitals. If it arrives near you, go and see it, not only for the beauty of the play, but also to enjoy the admiration and the curiosity of an audience when they discover, or rediscover, Freud and the genius of his imagination.

Chapter 8

A tribute to Bernardo Bertolucci[1]

In an interview a few years ago, Bernardo Bertolucci suggested that during the hour and forty minutes of the film's showing the viewer finds a way to sleep for ten minutes, and during those ten minutes to dream.

I don't believe I've ever been able to sleep, watching one of his films, but I have definitely dreamed a lot, starting from the time that I saw *Before the Revolution/Prima della Rivoluzione* (1964) in a theatre in my city, in the heart of Emilia (North Italy).

Many, many years have gone by since that time.

The deep feeling of that faraway Sunday afternoon of my adolescence has repeated itself many times, right up to when I saw his last work – those fifteen charming minutes of the short film *Histoire d'Eaux* (2002). It is an anecdote of time which wraps around itself, of contrasts which can capture in a single instant of awareness what happened in a minute, or in a year. It is as said in the lyrics sung by Mina, the famous Italian singer, in those years and in that short film: "and you will understand in a single moment what a year of love means."

In this long timespan I have never missed a chance to see a new Bertolucci film. Each time I have found something profound and something unique; something which would move me; something which would keep me company with a fragment of shared understanding; or something which stupefied me, which disturbed me, which consoled me – just as it should be with art and with beauty.

The cinema of Bertolucci has continued to offer me the chance to lose myself in my own memories, in an "Emilia"[2] which is dreamed of with music, melodrama, the real/unreal *piazze* (squares), the Sabbioneta/Tara of *The Spider's Stratagem/Strategia del Ragno* (1970b), magic in the hot fog of summer, a theatre of the unconscious in which the eternal conflict between fathers and sons is represented.

Or in the farmyard of *1900/Novecento*, overcrowded, busy with the faces and bodies of farmers at the border between the Middle Ages and modern times. And it simply doesn't matter that Olmo of *1900/Novecento* (1976) is the very-French Depardieu!

There, straddling between history and familiar myths, I could locate the same power as that of the uncles from my childhood. Their Herculean force had forced the retreat from the village of an entire fascist crowd which had gathered to punish them for their socialist sin, forcing castor oil down their throats. Those uncles who, after having threshed and harvested, would quench their thirst downing *lambrusco* by the bucketful.[3] Those uncles with pure Emilian names, like Athos Magnani of *The Spider's Stratagem/Strategia del Ragno*, even though fascism had taken the final "s" from one of my uncles' names, leaving him forever a surprised "Atho."[4] Well before having learned the real history, that was for me the discovery of a power which can violate any law, being one that can mutilate even your own name.

These are memories and with them comes the sense of loss, the pain of separation – a fundamental theme in the human psyche, which appears in every film by Bertolucci.

The traumatic loss of childhood's empire (*The Last Emperor/L'Ultimo Imperatore*, 1987) and separation from that world are found in his films too: the enchanting moon, the bike races made while perched on the big kids' handlebars, running along the riverbanks in the evening (*Luna/La Luna*, 1979), the mystery of the maternal face which we will never completely decipher.

And all of this comes with the introspective depth of his characters, enriched by the creative encounter with psychoanalysis and with a specific characteristic of his cinema not to saturate the story – that is, always to leave a door open because, just as Renoir said to the young Bertolucci, "you never know, something or someone could come in and bring with them beauty and wealth."

It is History with a capital "H," which Bertolucci spreads out before our eyes, with all the emotion and poetry of a world which is writing its own story (*1900/Novecento*).

And he does it with the incomparable gift of the narrator who knows how to condense and untangle onscreen decades of complex events starting from some particular, from an imperial ideogram, and ending up with a little poetic insect which captures our imagination and makes us live the monstrous menace history is to the lives of individuals.

History is often – in Bertolucci's cinema – a perverse nightmare, which returns in the form of Marxist or Fascist power, as we are in Italy or in China. *The Conformist/Il Conformista* (1970a) offered us again not only the drama of Italy in the 1930s, but also the drama of those years in which the film was made, with its terrorism and the strategy of tension, revolutionary dreams, and the adolescent illusion of a clean ideology as in *Before the Revolution/Prima della Rivoluzione* (1964) and in *The Dreamers* (2003).

In his films there is also the dream of following wanderlust, in search of elsewhere, following the irresistible attraction of other cultures. He gives us the Africa of *The Sheltering Sky* and *Besieged/L'Assedio* (1998), the orient of the *Last Emperor/Ultimo Imperatore* and *Little Buddha/Piccolo Buddha* (1993). (But doesn't the funny group of Buddhist monks who crowd around the little Buddha "Jesse" seem, as someone has written, like a group of affectionate old aunts who have just finished baking some treat or another?)

To discern your own roots, but not limit yourself by that from which you come, and to explore courageously your own private self; to go in search of an elsewhere, always a little nostalgic, suspended there on that threshold where you pause before departing, just before the changes of life, like Fabrizio and Gina in *Before the Revolution/Prima della Rivoluzione*: Bertolucci's cinema has reflected that which an entire generation was experiencing and experimenting in the realm of erotic intimacy, the couple's destiny, the agony of losing the ideals of love (*The Sheltering Sky, Last Tango in Paris/Ultimo Tango a Parigi* (1972), *Stealing Beauty/Io Ballo da Sola* (1996), *Besieged/L'Assedio; The Dreamers*).

In each of his films we discovered something which we would not have found so richly represented without his cinema, with his intuitive, poetic genius in showing us our limits and, at the same time, the explosive force with which one can find paths of freedom.

It is his limitless ability to dream and represent his dreams, and the indisputable beauty of his artistic vision which endow his vision of things and our vision of things with prospective breadth and depth.

I have spoken about my transference towards the cinema of Bertolucci, but I know I am not alone in this.

A young patient spies a book of interviews with Bertolucci on my desk. Without hesitating she begins by saying how much she loved *Stealing Beauty/Io Ballo da Sola* and the session solidifies clearly as never before her dream to be and to remain a nymph who dances in the virtual woods of the internet, safe from the anguish of having to confront the transition from being a young girl to becoming a woman. She is trying to slow down that change, not because – like the protagonist in *Stealing Beauty/Io Ballo da Sola* – she does not know her own father, but because she too cannot rewrite the scene of the sexual and sentimental encounter from which she was born, still permeated by violence and primitive monstrosities.

For this and for much more – which others have said better than I – I thank Bernardo Bertolucci from the depths of my heart. And I believe I express sentiments we all share.

Notes

1 Presented by the author on the occasion of the Award to Bernardo Bertolucci at the Psychoanalytic Congress of the Italian Psychoanalytic Society, Siena, 2006.
2 A region in North Italy.
3 A typical wine from that region of Italy, light and sparkling.
4 During the fascist dictatorship, every foreign form of language had to be abolished in honour of the Italian culture.

References

Bertolucci, Bernardo. (dir.) *Before the Revolution/Prima della Rivoluzione*. 1964. Italy: Cineriz. Film.

Bertolucci, Bernardo. (dir.) *The Conformist/Il Conformista*. 1970a. Italy: Mars Film, Marianne Productions, Maran Film. Film.

Bertolucci, Bernardo. (dir.) *The Spider's Strategy/Strategia del Ragno*. 1970b. Italy, France: Rai – Radiotelevisione italiana S.p.A. Film.

Bertolucci, Bernardo. (dir.) *Last Tango in Paris/Ultimo Tango a Parigi*. 1972. Italy, France: PEA, Les Productions Artistes Associés. Film.

Bertolucci, Bernardo. (dir.) *1900/Novecento*. 1976. Italy, France, Federal Republic of Germany: PEA, Les Productions Artistes Associés Artemis Film. Film.

Bertolucci, Bernardo. (dir.) *La Luna*. 1979. Italy, USA: 20th Century Fox. Film.

Bertolucci, Bernardo. (dir.) *The Last Emperor/L'Ultimo Imperatore*. 1987. UK, Italy, China: Hemdale Film Corporation, Recorded Picture Company. Film.

Bertolucci, Bernardo. (dir.) *The Sheltering Sky*. 1990. UK, USA, Italy: Warner Bros. Canada. Film.

Bertolucci, Bernardo. (dir.) *Little Buddha/Il Piccolo Buddha*. 1993. UK, Italy, France: CiBy 2000, Serpcor Anstalt, Recorded Picture Company, Sahara Company. Film.

Bertolucci, Bernardo. (dir.) *Stealing Beauty/Io Ballo da Sola*. 1996. Italy: Fiction srl, Recorded Picture Company, UGC Images. Film.

Bertolucci, Bernardo. (dir.) *Besieged/L'Assedio*. 1998. Italy: Fiction, Navert Film, Mediaset. Film.

Bertolucci, Bernardo. (dir.) *Histoire d'Eaux*. 2002. Italy, Germany, UK: VIMEO. Film.

Bertolucci, Bernardo. (dir.) *The Dreamers*. 2003. UK, France, Italy: Recorded Picture. Film.

Index

Note: page numbers containing n refer to notes.

For Product Safety Concerns and Information please contact our EU representative GPSR@taylorandfrancis.com Taylor & Francis Verlag GmbH, Kaufingerstraße 24, 80331 München, Germany